Integrated Behavioral Health in Pediatric Practice

Editors

ROGER W. APPLE
CHERYL A. DICKSON
MARIA DEMMA I. CABRAL

PEDIATRIC CLINICS
OF NORTH AMERICA

www.pediatric.theclinics.com

Consulting Editor
BONITA F. STANTON

June 2021 • Volume 68 • Number 3

ELSEVIER

1600 John F. Kennedy Boulevard • Suite 1800 • Philadelphia, Pennsylvania, 19103-2899

http://www.theclinics.com

THE PEDIATRIC CLINICS OF NORTH AMERICA Volume 68, Number 3
June 2021 ISSN 0031-3955, ISBN-13: 978-0-323-83596-1

Editor: Kerry Holland
Developmental Editor: Axell Ivan Jade M. Purificacion

The Pediatric Clinics of North America (ISSN 0031-3955) is published bimonthly by Elsevier Inc., 360 Park Avenue South, New York, NY 10010-1710. Months of issue are February, April, June, August, October, and December. Periodicals postage paid at New York, NY and additional mailing offices. Subscription prices are $250.00 per year (US individuals), $984.00 per year (US institutions), $315.00 per year (Canadian individuals), $1048.00 per year (Canadian institutions), $376.00 per year (international individuals), $1048.00 per year (international institutions), $100.00 per year (US students and residents), $100.00 per year (Canadian students and residents), and $165.00 per year (international residents and students). To receive students/resident rare, orders must be accompanied by name of affiliated institution, date of term, and the signature of program/residency coordinator on institution letterhead. Orders will be billed at individual rate until proof of status is received. Foreign air speed delivery is included in all *Clinics* subscription prices. All prices are subject to change without notice. **POSTMASTER:** Send address changes to *The Pediatric Clinics of North America*, Elsevier Health Sciences Division, Subscription Customer Service, 3251 Riverport Lane, Maryland Heights, MO 63043. **Customer Service: 1-800-654-2452 (US and Canada). From outside of the US and Canada: 1-314-447-8871. Fax: 1-314-447-8029. For print support, E-mail: JournalsCustomerService-usa@elsevier. com. For online support, E-mail: JournalsOnlineSupport-usa@elsevier.com.**

Reprints. For copies of 100 or more, of articles in this publication, please contact the Commercial Reprints Department, Elsevier Inc., 360 Park Avenue South, New York, NY 10010-1710. Tel.: 212-633-3874; Fax: 212-633-3820; E-mail: reprints@elsevier.com.

The Pediatric Clinics of North America is also published in Spanish by McGraw-Hill Inter-americana Editores S.A., Mexico City, Mexico; in Portuguese by Riechmann and Affonso Editores, Rua Comandante Coelho 1085, CEP 21250, Rio de Janeiro, Brazil; and in Greek by Althayia SA, Athens, Greece.

The Pediatric Clinics of North America is covered in *MEDLINE/PubMed (Index Medicus)*, *Excerpta Medica*, *Current Contents, Current Contents/Clinical Medicine, Science Citation Index, ASCA, ISI/BIOMED*, and *BIOSIS*.

PROGRAM OBJECTIVE

The goal of the *Pediatric Clinics of North America* is to keep practicing physicians and residents up to date with current clinical practice in pediatrics by providing timely articles reviewing the state-of-the-art in patient care.

TARGET AUDIENCE

All practicing pediatricians, physicians and healthcare professionals who provide patient care to pediatric patients.

LEARNING OBJECTIVES

Upon completion of this activity, participants will be able to:

1. Review basic concepts of Integrated Behavioral Health (IBH) in pediatric practice as an intervention model.
2. Discuss the most common pediatric psychological and behavioral concerns that present in different health settings.
3. Recognize the utility of remote consultation and telemedicine platforms in the delivery of IBH services.

ACCREDITATIONS

Physician Credit

The Elsevier Office of Continuing Medical Education (EOCME) is accredited by the Accreditation Council for Continuing Medical Education (ACCME) to provide continuing medical education for physicians.

The EOCME designates this journal-based activity for a maximum of 15 *AMA PRA Category 1 Credit*(s)™. Physicians should claim only the credit commensurate with the extent of their participation in the activity.

All other healthcare professionals requesting continuing education credit for this this journal-based activity will be issued a certificate of participation.

ABP Maintenance of Certification Credit

Successful completion of this CME activity, which includes participation in the activity and individual assessment of and feedback to the learner, enables the learner to earn up to 15 MOC points in the American Board of Pediatrics' (ABP) Maintenance of Certification (MOC) program. It is the CME activity provider's responsibility to submit learner completion information to ACCME for the purpose of granting ABP MOC credit.

DISCLOSURE OF CONFLICTS OF INTEREST

The EOCME assesses conflict of interest with its instructors, faculty, planners, and other individuals who are in a position to control the content of CME activities. All relevant conflicts of interest that are identified are thoroughly vetted by EOCME for fair balance, scientific objectivity, and patient care recommendations. EOCME is committed to providing its learners with CME activities that promote improvements or quality in healthcare and not a specific proprietary business or a commercial interest.

The planning committee, staff, authors and editors listed below have identified no financial relationships or relationships to products or devices they or their spouse/life partner have with commercial interest related to the content of this CME activity:
Sonia Amin, PhD; Roger W. Apple, PhD; Mark S. Barajas, PhD; Swati Y. Bhave, MD, MBBS, DCH; Derrick Bines, PhD; Maria Demma Cabral, MD; Jessica Campbell, BS; Kevin Cates, MD; Summer S. Chahin, MA; Regina Chavous-Gibson, MSN, RN; Ethel Clemente, MD; Pilar Corcoran-Lozano, MA; Parker Crutchfield, PhD; Jocelyn DeLeon, MD; Cheryl Dickson, MD, MPH; Nicole Fledderman, MD; Scott T. Gaynor, PhD; Tyler S. Gibb, JD, PhD; Kristine M. Gibson, MD, FAAP; Donald E. Greydanus, MD; Kerry Holland; Khadijah Hussain, BS; Heidi Joshi, PsyD; Gordon Liu; Sheryl Lozowski-Sullivan, MPH, PhD; Skye Lu, DO; Rajkumar Mayakrishnann; Rajesh Mehta, MD; John Minser, MFA; Theron O'Halloran, MD; Dilip R. Patel, MBBS, MBA, MPH; Keshav Patel, MS; Harish K. Pemde, MD, FIAP; Rachel A. Petts, PhD; Jessica Ramsay; Michael J. Redinger, MD, MA; Neelkamal Soares, MD; Lydia Stetson, MA; Jason Straussman, MSW; Alexander W. Sullivan, BA; Joshua VandeBurgh, MD; Katie White, MA

UNAPPROVED/OFF-LABEL USE DISCLOSURE

The EOCME requires CME faculty to disclose to the participants:

1. When products or procedures being discussed are off-label, unlabelled, experimental, and/or investigational (not US Food and Drug Administration [FDA] approved); and

2. Any limitations on the information presented, such as data that are preliminary or that represent ongoing research, interim analyses, and/or unsupported opinions. Faculty may discuss information about pharmaceutical agents that is outside of FDA-approved labelling. This information is intended solely for CME and is not intended to promote off-label use of these medications. If you have any questions, contact the medical affairs department of the manufacturer for the most recent prescribing information.

TO ENROLL

To enroll in the *Pediatric Clinics of North America* Continuing Medical Education program, call customer service at 1-800-654-2452 or sign up online at http://www.theclinics.com/home/cme. The CME program is available to subscribers for an additional annual fee of USD 324.00.

METHOD OF PARTICIPATION

In order to claim credit, participants must complete the following:
1. Complete enrolment as indicated above.
2. Read the activity.
3. Complete the CME Test and Evaluation. Participants must achieve a score of 70% on the test. All CME Tests and Evaluations must be completed online.

In order to claim MOC points, participants must complete the following:
1. Complete steps listed above for claiming CME credit
2. Provide your specialty board ID#, birth date (MM/DD), and attestation.
3. Online MOC submission is only available for the American Board of pediatrics' (ABP) Maintenance of Certification (MOC) program

CME INQUIRIES/SPECIAL NEEDS

For all CME inquiries or special needs, please contact elsevierCME@elsevier.com

Contributors

CONSULTING EDITOR

BONITA F. STANTON, MD
Founding Dean, Robert C. and Laura C. Garrett Endowed Chair, Hackensack Meridian School of Medicine, President, Academic Enterprise, Hackensack Meridian Health, Nutley, New Jersey, USA

EDITORS

ROGER W. APPLE, PhD
Associate Professor, Division Chief, Pediatric Psychology, Director, WMed Health Pediatric Autism Center, Department of Pediatric and Adolescent Medicine, Western Michigan University Homer Stryker M.D. School of Medicine, Kalamazoo, Michigan, USA

CHERYL A. DICKSON, MD, MPH
Associate Professor of Pediatrics, Department of Pediatric and Adolescent Medicine, Associate Dean, Health Equity and Community Affairs, Western Michigan University Homer Stryker M.D. School of Medicine, Kalamazoo, Michigan, USA

MARIA DEMMA I. CABRAL, MD
Associate Professor, Division Chief, Department of Pediatric and Adolescent Medicine, Western Michigan University Homer Stryker M.D. School of Medicine, Kalamazoo, Michigan, USA

AUTHORS

SONIA AMIN, PhD
Post-Doctoral Fellow in Health Service Psychology, University of California, Berkeley, Berkeley, California, USA

ROGER W. APPLE, PhD
Associate Professor, Division Chief, Pediatric Psychology, Director, WMed Health Pediatric Autism Center, Department of Pediatric and Adolescent Medicine, Western Michigan University Homer Stryker M.D. School of Medicine, Kalamazoo, Michigan, USA

MARK S. BARAJAS, PhD
Associate Professor and Licensed Psychologist, Department of Psychology, Saint Mary's College of California, Moraga, California, USA

SWATI Y. BHAVE, MD, DCH, FCPS, FIAP, FAAP (HON)
Executive Director, AACCI, Association of Adolescent and Child Care in India, Mumbai, India; Adjunct Professor in Adolescent Medicine, Dr D.Y. Patil Medical College, Pimpri, India; Dr D.Y. Patil Vidyapeeth, Pune, India

DERRICK BINES, PhD
Assistant Professor, Department of Counseling, San Francisco State University, San Francisco, California, USA

MARIA DEMMA I. CABRAL, MD
Associate Professor, Division Chief, Department of Pediatric and Adolescent Medicine, Western Michigan University Homer Stryker M.D. School of Medicine, Kalamazoo, Michigan, USA

JESSICA CAMPBELL, BS
Pediatric Psychology Subspecialty, Department of Pediatric and Adolescent Medicine, Western Michigan University Homer Stryker M.D. School of Medicine, Western Michigan University, Kalamazoo, Michigan, USA

KEVIN CATES, MD, MPH
Harvard South Shore Psychiatry Residency, Brockton, Massachusetts, USA

SUMMER S. CHAHIN, MA
Division of Pediatric Psychology, Western Michigan University, Western Michigan University Homer Stryker M.D. School of Medicine, Kalamazoo, Michigan, USA

ETHEL CLEMENTE, MD
Assistant Professor, Department of Pediatric and Adolescent Medicine, Western Michigan University Homer Stryker M.D. School of Medicine, Kalamazoo, Michigan, USA

PILAR CORCORAN-LOZANO, MA
John F. Kennedy University, John F. Kennedy School of Psychology at National University, Pleasant Hill, California, USA

PARKER CRUTCHFIELD, PhD
Associate Professor, Program in Medical Ethics, Humanities and Law, Western Michigan University Homer Stryker M.D. School of Medicine, Kalamazoo, Michigan, USA

JOCELYN DELEON, MD
Assistant Professor, Department of Pediatric and Adolescent Medicine, Western Michigan University Homer Stryker M.D. School of Medicine, Kalamazoo, Michigan, USA

CHERYL A. DICKSON, MD, MPH
Associate Professor of Pediatrics, Department of Pediatric and Adolescent Medicine, Associate Dean, Health Equity and Community Affairs, Western Michigan University Homer Stryker M.D. School of Medicine, Kalamazoo, Michigan, USA

NICOLE FLEDDERMAN, MD
Department of Pediatric and Adolescent Medicine, Western Michigan University Homer Stryker M.D. School of Medicine, Kalamazoo, Michigan, USA

SCOTT T. GAYNOR, PhD
Professor, Department of Psychology, Western Michigan University, Kalamazoo, Michigan, USA

TYLER S. GIBB, JD, PhD
Assistant Professor, Co-Chief, Program in Medical Ethics, Humanities and Law, Western Michigan University Homer Stryker M.D. School of Medicine, Kalamazoo, Michigan, USA

KRISTINE M. GIBSON, MD, FAAP
Assistant Dean for Clinical Applications, Assistant Professor of Pediatric and Adolescent Medicine, Western Michigan University Homer Stryker M.D. School of Medicine, Kalamazoo, Michigan, USA

DONALD E. GREYDANUS, MD, DrHC (Athens)
Professor, Department of Pediatric and Adolescent Medicine, Western Michigan University Homer Stryker M.D. School of Medicine, Kalamazoo, Michigan, USA

KHADIJAH HUSSAIN, BS
Medical Student, MD Candidate Class of 2022, Western Michigan University Homer Stryker M.D. School of Medicine, Kalamazoo, Michigan, USA

HEIDI JOSHI, PsyD
Behavioral Health Program Manager, John Muir Health Family Medicine Residency, Walnut Creek, California, USA

GORDON LIU, BA
Medical Student, Western Michigan University Homer Stryker M.D. School of Medicine, Kalamazoo, Michigan, USA

SHERYL LOZOWSKI-SULLIVAN, MPH, PhD
Clinical Psychologist, Department of Pediatric and Adolescent Medicine, Western Michigan University Homer Stryker M.D. School of Medicine, Kalamazoo, Michigan, USA

SKYE LU, DO
Primary Care Pediatrician, Yu Pediatrics, Colonial Heights, Virginia, USA

RAJESH MEHTA, MD
Regional Advisor, Neonatal, Child and Adolescent Health, WHO South East Asia, New Delhi, India

JOHN MINSER, MFA
Instructor, Program in Medical Ethics, Humanities and Law, Western Michigan University Homer Stryker M.D. School of Medicine, Kalamazoo, Michigan, USA

THERON O'HALLORAN, MD
Western Michigan University Homer Stryker M.D. School of Medicine, Kalamazoo, Michigan, USA

DILIP R. PATEL, MBBS, MBA, MPH
Department Chair and Professor, Department of Pediatric and Adolescent Medicine, Western Michigan University Homer Stryker M.D. School of Medicine, Kalamazoo, Michigan, USA

KESHAV PATEL, MS
Pediatric Psychology Subspecialty, Department of Pediatric and Adolescent Medicine, Western Michigan University Homer Stryker M.D. School of Medicine, Kalamazoo, Michigan, USA

HARISH K. PEMDE, MD, FIAP
Director, Professor, Department of Pediatrics, Head, WHO Collaborating Center for Training and Research in Adolescent Health, Lady Hardinge Medical College, Kalawati Saran Children's Hospital, New Delhi, India

RACHEL A. PETTS, PhD
Assistant Professor, Department of Psychology, Wichita State University, Wichita, Kansas, USA

JESSICA RAMSAY, MD
Western Michigan University Homer Stryker M.D. School of Medicine, Kalamazoo, Michigan

MICHAEL J. REDINGER, MD, MA
Assistant Professor, Department of Psychiatry, Co-Chief, Program in Medical Ethics, Humanities and Law, Western Michigan University Homer Stryker M.D. School of Medicine, Kalamazoo, Michigan, USA

NEELKAMAL SOARES, MD
Developmental-Behavioral Pediatrician, Faculty, Western Michigan University Homer Stryker M.D. School of Medicine, Kalamazoo, Michigan, USA

LYDIA STETSON, MA
MA Instructor, Division of Pediatric Psychology, Western Michigan University Homer Stryker M.D. School of Medicine, Kalamazoo, Michigan, USA

JASON STRAUSSMAN, MSW
Clinical Social Worker, Tang Counseling Center, University of California, Berkeley, Berkeley, California, USA

ALEXANDER W. SULLIVAN, BA
MSW Candidate, Department of Social Work, Wayne State University, Detroit, Michigan, USA

JOSHUA VANDEBURGH, MD
PGY -1 Neurology Resident, University of Minnesota, Minneapolis, Minnesota, USA

KATIE WHITE, MA
Assistant Professor, Division of Pediatric Psychology, Western Michigan University Homer Stryker M.D. School of Medicine, Kalamazoo, Michigan, USA

Contents

Most children and adolescents with behavioral and mental health concerns first present to their pediatricians. Although pediatricians are fully cognizant of the importance of addressing behavioral and mental health concerns, they often find it difficult to deliver such care effectively and efficiently within a typical practice setting. Integration of medical and behavioral health care has emerged as a model to deliver such care. In the pediatric primary care practice, integrated behavioral health has been shown to be a cost-effective way to deliver high-quality care. This article describes basic definitions and contexts of integrated pediatric behavioral health.

Humans have long sought to be provided with optimal health care, and the research continues in the twenty-first century. In the spirit of Galen from 19 centuries ago, empowering the patient's physician remains an important approach in health care. There is an emphasis on primary care and integration of behavioral consultation services in primary care. It remains a work in progress with help from the past and realistic hope for the future.

Children and adolescents with clinically concerning behavioral health conditions face several barriers to accessing specialized mental health care. One proposed solution is to improve and expand integrated care provided in the primary health care provider's office. Several strategies can increase pediatrician comfort and willingness to collaborate in diagnosing and treating behavioral health conditions, and increased utilization of new technologies (such as telehealth) are likely to play an increasingly important role in the process.

established programs have been in existence for childhood cancer and
cystic fibrosis.

The integrated behavioral health care model in primary care has the potential to reduce barriers to care experienced by children and families from
ethnic minorities and low socioeconomic status. Limited access to pediatric behavioral health care is a significant problem, with up to 40% of children and adolescents with identified mental disorders and only 30% of
them receiving care. Barriers include transportation, insurance, and
shortage of specialists. Primary care provider bias, decreased knowledge
and feelings of competence, and cultural beliefs and stigma also affect
earlier diagnosis and treatment, particularly for Hispanic families with
low English proficiency and African Americans.

Pediatric patients often work with multiple health care providers for complex presenting concerns. This complexity has called for pediatric health
care providers to strengthen interdisciplinary relationships with mental
health providers to meet patient needs. Integrated behavioral health
collaborative practice models, using the Interprofessional Education
Collaborative competencies, provide the necessary scaffolding to train
medical and mental health professionals. A multicultural framework can
be integrated into the interprofessional education curricula to better equip
health care professionals to provide culturally competent services that de-
center hierarchy, power, privilege, and implicit bias, resulting in improved
access and quality of comprehensive health care services.

Accumulating evidence documenting the high percentage of patients who
first discuss mental health needs with their primary care physician has
accelerated the integration of physical and mental health care to a national
priority. Several models have been developed describing how health care
settings can integrate physical and mental health care and how training
programs might better prepare clinicians to work in integrated behavioral
health care settings. This article explores models of integrated behavioral
health, highlights contributions of social work and psychology, and describes the training and experiences of social workers and psychologists
working in integrated behavioral health.

This article explores the role of assessments in integrated behavioral health within a pediatric primary care setting, specifically exploring what valid and reliable standardized assessments may be used and for what concerns the assessment be of most use. The article also considers how assessments used by integrated behavioral health may inform the type of evidenced-based intervention that would be most appropriate and efficacious for the patient, as well as assist in determining if longer term or more formal mental health treatment may be required.

PEDIATRIC CLINICS OF NORTH AMERICA

SERIES OF RELATED INTEREST

Clinics in Perinatology
http://www.perinatology.theclinics.com/
Advances in Pediatrics
http://www.advancesinpediatrics.com/

THE CLINICS ARE AVAILABLE ONLINE!
Access your subscription at:
www.theclinics.com

Foreword

Integrating General Child Health Care and Mental Health Care in Pediatric Primary Care Settings

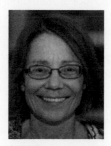

Bonita F. Stanton, MD
Consulting Editor

Since the end of the twentieth century, recognition of the importance of integrating behavioral health into both child and adult primary care has been growing. There are myriad reasons for such integration, including the high frequency of behavioral conditions in the general population and the greater likelihood that for reasons of convenience, cost, and privacy, families would seek care in the same office at which they receive their general care.[1]

Despite the fact that these conditions are prevalent in all age groups, to date, children have received less treatment and research focus than have adults. A preponderance of the research on behavioral health integration has focused on adults, despite the substantial prevalence of these disorders among children. For example, while an estimated 13% to 20% of children in the United States have been diagnosed with a mental disorder, the supply of pediatric mental health specialists appears to be inadequate among virtually all states, with over 40 estimated to have a severe shortage.[2]

Fortunately for our nation's children, the situation appears to be changing. In recent years, there has been an increase in collaborative efforts between pediatricians and pediatric psychologists, leading to greater availability of services and better integrated care models. Nevertheless, there is still substantial variation in the behavioral models driving the intervention approaches, and therefore, in the outcomes and clinical guidelines. As these collaborations have grown in recent years and have led to research collaborations, data regarding their effectiveness have become available. One such study involving over 4000children found that approximately two-thirds of children seen for well-child visits in an urban, largely publicly insured population also received behavioral health services, leading to recommendations and medical diagnoses. The authors conclude that when such services are provided, the families do seek them, but acknowledge that privacy and cost remain barriers. Models exist, however, for treating many of these children effectively in primary care settings that offer integrated, family-centered care.[3,4]

This issue of *Pediatric Clinics of North America* seeks to guide pediatricians, child mental health professionals, and other child health care providers who are looking for research-supported models of behavioral health integration that will improve the health of children with mental disorders.

Bonita F. Stanton, MD
Hackensack Meridian School of Medicine
Academic Enterprise
Hackensack Meridian Health
Hackensack Meridian School of Medicine
123 Metro Boulevard
Nutley, NJ 07110, USA

E-mail address:
bonita.stanton@hmhn.org

REFERENCES

1. Kolko DJ, Perrin E. The integration of behavioral health interventions in children's health care services: services, science, and suggestions. J Child Adolesc Psychol 2014;43(2):216–28.
2. Tyler ETT, Hulkower RL, Kamiinski JW. Behavioral health integration in pediatric primary care: considerations and opportunities for policymakers, planners and providers. Milbank Memorial Fund. 2017. Available at: www.milbank.org. https://www.researchgate.net/publication/315665118. Accessed April 13, 2021.
3. Stancin T, Perrin EC. Psychologists and pediatricians: opportunities for collaboration in primary care. Am Psychol 2014;69(4):332–43.
4. Talmi A, Muther EF, Margolis K, et al. The scope of behavioral health integration in a pediatric primary care setting. J Pediatr Psychol 2016;41(10):1120–32.

Preface

Integrated Behavioral Health in Pediatric Practice

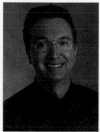 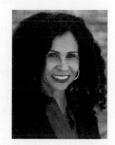 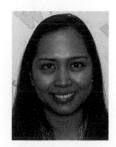

Roger W. Apple, PhD   Cheryl A. Dickson, MD, MPH   Maria Demma I. Cabral, MD
Editors

Children and adolescents with psychological concerns often first present to their pediatric provider; however, many pediatric practices are not equipped to adequately address the challenges, stressors, and psychological and behavioral problems that commonly occur in children and adolescents. Proper inquiry of related issues that leads to disclosure and provision of mental and behavioral health care is expected to occur. However, despite the obvious demand, limited or lack of knowledge, comfort level, resources, and access create gaps in delivery of services that are not always readily available. Integrated Behavioral Health (IBH) services staffed by psychologists help fill these gaps in care in a coordinated and collaborative manner and have shown great promise in the field of pediatrics.

This focused issue of *Pediatric Clinics of North America* on IBH in Pediatric Practice conveys the basic concepts of IBH from a historical perspective to its continuum as an intervention model, in both the primary and subspecialty pediatric clinical settings. Awareness of the most common psychological and behavioral concerns that present in different health settings is crucial in the conceptualization and implementation of IBH. The IBH behavior consultant assists with the use of brief screening tools or formal assessments and helps identify applicable intervention strategies. The on-site availability of IBH services that allows for care delivery at the time of identification of problems helps mitigate the stigma associated with psychological and behavioral health disorders. With operational challenges, such as distance from the clinic or the given current times of the coronavirus pandemic, IBH services can be utilized with remote consultation and treatment by telemedicine platforms. The role of the behavioral consultant goes beyond patient care, with emphasis on educating and training willing and committed health care providers. Adaptation of IBH care delivery allows for interprofessional collaboration and early career trainee introduction.

Pediatr Clin N Am 68 (2021) xvii–xviii
https://doi.org/10.1016/j.pcl.2021.03.002
0031-3955/21/© 2021 Published by Elsevier Inc.

pediatric.theclinics.com

The fruition of our focused issues is a collaborative work from different specialists, bringing enriching perspectives in the field of IBH. Our common goal is to provide readers current, practical, and applicable information for the health care provider, especially pediatricians, who recognize the vast need to promote and deliver a conscious and effective patient-centered treatment.

Roger W. Apple, PhD
Department of Pediatric and
Adolescent Medicine
Western Michigan University
Homer Stryker M.D. School of Medicine
1000 Oakland Drive
Kalamazoo, MI 49008, USA

Cheryl A. Dickson, MD, MPH
Department of Pediatric and
Adolescent Medicine
Western Michigan University
Homer Stryker MD School of Medicine
1000 Oakland Drive
Kalamazoo, MI 49008, USA

Maria Demma I. Cabral, MD
Department of Pediatric and
Adolescent Medicine
Western Michigan University
Homer Stryker MD School of Medicine
1000 Oakland Drive
Kalamazoo, MI 49008, USA

E-mail addresses:
roger.apple@med.wmich.edu (R.W. Apple)
Cheryl.dickson@med.wmich.edu (C.A. Dickson)
mariademma.cabral@med.wmich.edu (M.D.I. Cabral)

Integrated Behavioral Health: Definitions and Contexts

Nicole Fledderman, MD*, Jocelyn DeLeon, MD,
Dilip R. Patel, MBBS, MBA, MPH

KEYWORDS

- Integrated behavioral health (IBH) • Pediatric • Behavioral health • Primary care
- Mental health care

KEY POINTS

- Most children and adolescents with behavioral and mental health concerns first present to their pediatricians; however, pediatricians have often found it difficult to deliver such care effectively within a typical practice setting.
- Integrating mental and behavioral health care with primary care can lower the costs of care and improve the quality of patient care.
- Integrated behavioral health is defined as primary care providers and behavioral and mental health care providers working together to provide comprehensive health care in a cost-effective way
- Different models of integrated behavioral health care represent an increasing level of integration between primary care and behavioral health.

INTRODUCTION

Most children with behavioral and mental health conditions initially present in a pediatric primary care setting. The World Health Organization defines mental health as "a state of well-being in which every individual realizes his or her own potential, can cope with the normal stresses of life, can work productively and fruitfully, and is able to make a contribution to her or his community."[1] It is infrequent for children and adolescents with behavioral and mental health conditions to first present in the specialized mental health care practice.[2,3] An estimated 50% of mental health disorders have their onset by the age of 14 years.[2,3] Failure to recognize behavioral or mental health concerns early and suboptimal treatment have been associated with significant long-term adverse outcomes.[3,4] When compared with the general population, persons with severe mental illness often die 13 to 30 years early.[3] Most of these early deaths can be

Department of Pediatric and Adolescent Medicine, Western Michigan University Homer Stryker M.D. School of Medicine, 1000 Oakland Drive, Kalamazoo, MI 49008, USA
* Corresponding author.
E-mail address: nicole.fledderman@med.wmich.edu

Pediatr Clin N Am 68 (2021) 511–518
https://doi.org/10.1016/j.pcl.2021.02.007
pediatric.theclinics.com
0031-3955/21/© 2021 Elsevier Inc. All rights reserved.

prevented by early recognition and optimal treatment of mental illness. It is difficult for a typical pediatric practice to deliver behavioral and mental health care effectively and efficiently without collaboration with mental health services.[3] Combining mental health services with primary care can reduce costs, increase the quality of care, and ultimately save lives.[3] Integrated behavioral health (IBH) is defined as primary care providers (PCP) and behavioral and mental health care providers working together to provide comprehensive health care in a cost-effective way.

Behavioral health, when practiced within the context of the pediatric primary medical care setting, reflects some level of integration between the two. Because most children and adolescents with behavioral health concerns are initially seen in a primary care setting, it is useful to have an understanding of what is considered primary medical care, especially in the United States. There has been a relentless discussion of primary care in the United States on a daily basis in the scientific and lay media and various other venues of discourse. Many experts contend that primary care, or lack thereof, is the most important aspect of the health care system that must be addressed to save or rescue the US health care system from impending catastrophe.

PRIMARY CARE

In 1961, White and colleagues[5] first used the term "primary medical care" in their work on the ecology of medical care. The World Health Organization, in 1978, following an international conference in Alma-Ata, Kazakhstan, elaborated on the need and role of primary health care.[6] Primary care, or primary medical care, is considered the most critical component of health care delivery in the United States. Kovner and colleagues[7] have cited several reasons for this: primary care provides the initial point of contact for individuals seeking medical care, primary care practitioners are essential in coordination of patient care within the health care system, primary care practitioners are able to effectively engage the patient and family in promoting their health, and evidence suggests that increased access to primary care improves quality of care and reduces cost of care. Starfield and colleagues[8] in their extensive review have also discussed the rationale and benefits of primary care for health, which includes greater access to needed services, better quality of care, a greater focus on prevention, early management of health problems, the cumulative effect of the main primary care delivery characteristics, and the role of primary care in reducing unnecessary and potentially harmful specialist care.

A widely cited definition of primary care is that proposed by the Institute of Medicine[9,10]: "Primary care is the provision of integrated, accessible health care services by clinicians who are accountable for addressing a large majority of personal health care needs, developing a sustained partnership with patients, and practicing in the context of family and community."

According to Goroll and Mulley,[11] each of the definitions of primary care has evolved within the historical context at the time. Within the context of the current health care system in the United States, the most predominant definition of primary care is based on functional attributes of the primary care system of care.[11] Goroll and Mulley[11] have provided the following definitions of primary care:

- Systems Definition: The systems definition of primary care integrates the attributes of site of first contact for the patient and the continuity of care.
- Task-Oriented Definition: Another way of defining primary care is a definition based on the work of a primary care clinician. Task-oriented definition includes the following key tasks within the context of primary care: integrating medical and psychological diagnosis and treatment; eliciting and responding to patient

attributions, requests, and preferences; mastering the use and interpretation of diagnostic tests; interpreting the medical literature and applying it to the care of individual patients; attending to the patient's social network; and planning for end-of-life care.

- Function-Oriented Definition: Includes the first contact, longitudinal, continuous, comprehensive, and coordinated care.
- A Cross-Disciplinary Academic Definition: The cross-disciplinary academic definition encompasses the research and educational domains of primary care. This definition evolved from interdisciplinary research, predominantly with social sciences and includes such other areas with impact on health as economics, communication, epidemiology, and biostatistics.
- Professional Definition: This definition is similar to those used by some of the government agencies and organized medicine. It recognizes formal medical specialties of family medicine, general internal medicine, pediatrics, obstetrics and gynecology, and other self-designated specialties. The essential characteristic of professional definition of primary care is that the practitioners define their own scope of primary care practice.

CHARACTERISTICS OF INTEGRATED HEALTH CARE

The basic characteristics of integrated health care are coordination, continuity, and its comprehensive scope. Both major aspects of integrated health care (care coordination and care continuum) are comprehensive in that they span across different providers, different health care delivery settings, and different levels or intensity of medical care delivered.[12–14]

Continuity of medical care should occur on a longitudinal basis, and ideally over the life span of the individual. Continuity of care encompasses the care provided by the same health care provider and the same interprofessional team of providers over time.

Coordination of medical care includes timely and efficient sharing of relevant information between providers and different services including community-based agencies. Communication between providers and agencies in a timely manner is an essential characteristic of integrated health care. Individuals should be able to access care when needed and any barriers to care should be addressed, including administrative, financial, or sociocultural.

DEFINITION OF INTEGRATED BEHAVIORAL HEALTH

The Lexicon for Behavioral Health and Primary Care Integration, recently published by the Agency for Healthcare Research and Quality, defines integrated behavioral health care as follows[13]:

The care that results from a practice team of primary care and behavioral health clinicians, working together with patients and families, using a systematic and cost-effective approach to provide patient-centered care for a defined population. This care may address mental health and substance abuse conditions, health behaviors (including their contribution to chronic medical illnesses), life stressors and crises, stress-related physical symptoms, and ineffective patterns of health care utilization.

Behavioral health can be applied broadly as an integral part of any medical care. The practice of behavioral health in an integrated model addresses not only behavioral symptoms but also multiple psychological and behavioral factors that are associated with acute or chronic illness.[14]

The core principles of the IBH model are applicable across all age groups.[3,12,13] Ongoing social, psychological, and cognitive development in children and adolescents is an essential differentiating consideration when applying IBH principles to the care of children and adolescents, especially those with complex medical conditions.[3] When compared with adults, the application and delivery of IBH in the pediatric practice setting differs in three key aspects: (1) sensitivity to social, emotional, and psychological development; (2) the essential role of family and other caregivers; and (3) greater importance of coping strategy and adjustment in treatment plan.[3,12,13] Intellectual disability and developmental delay should be considered as part of the evaluation of children and adolescents who have behavioral concerns.[3] In a pediatric setting, normal or typical behaviors of children and adolescents as these relate to health-related lifestyle should also be considered. Behavioral health also includes mental health conditions seen in children and adolescents, which may be recognized as primary concerns or in association with acute or chronic medical conditions.[14–16]

IBH is patient-centered in that it respects the participation of the patient in making informed choices related to his or her health or medical care. Collaboration among the patient, family, and health care team is an essential characteristic of IBH.

Integration of care by its nature implies a systems-level approach to care delivery. It is not necessary for all the team members to be physically in the same place to deliver integrated care. Different models of IBH have been described (**Table 1**).[3,13,16] These models exist along a spectrum of progressively higher level of integration between medical and behavioral health care.

MODELS OF INTEGRATED BEHAVIORAL HEALTH CARE
Coordinated

Coordinated IBH model is at the lower end of the spectrum of integration. They key characteristic of this model is effective interdisciplinary communication, which includes sharing of relevant health-related information between the pediatrician and behavioral health consultant.[3,13,14] Increasingly, telephone consultations with child psychiatrists and pediatric psychologists by pediatricians is becoming a common practice. Pediatricians are able to consult with a behavioral health specialist over the telephone regarding appropriate intervention and treatment. Sometimes this method can involve care coordinators who serve as the intermediary between physicians and mental health providers. This model is cost effective compared with hiring full time behavioral health consultants by the practice. In a coordinated model, different professional disciplines are not necessarily located in the same practice setting.

Colocated

In colocated IBH model, the pediatric primary care and behavioral health service are located in the same practice setting. However, each practice operates functionally independent of each other; patients with need are referred from the pediatric to the behavioral health service.[3,13,16] Colocation describes where care is being provided rather than indicating a collaboration between providers regarding the patient's treatment plan (each provider has separate treatment plans).[13] Being located in the same setting provides an excellent resource to the pediatrician and behavioral health consultant being able to access each other and consult when necessary.[13,16] A potential benefit of colocated services is sharing the same electronic medical record, effectively increasing access to information.

Table 1
Comparison of key features of different models of integrated behavioral health care

Features	Model			
Key Element	Coordinated Care	Colocated Care	Collaborative/Fully Integrated	Primary Care Behavioral Health
	Communication	Physical Proximity	Practice Change	Practice Change
Where is care provided?	Separate facilities	In same facility not necessarily same offices	In the same space in the same facility (some to all of the space is shared)	In the same space in the same facility (some to all of the space is shared)
Electronic medical record	Separate systems	May have separate systems or may share some systems	Shared system	Shared system
Treatment plan	Separate treatment plans	Separate plans may be informed by shared information; collaborative treatment planning for specific patients	Collaborative treatment planning for all shared patients	Collaborative treatment planning for all patients
Level of communication/interaction	Low; primarily triggered by referral/consultation; communication rarely occurs in person	Partial; curbside consultation; meet occasionally to coordinate plans for specific patients; communication may occur in person or via telephone or e-mail	Complete; regular in person communication; have regular team meetings to discuss overall patient care and specific patient issues	Complete
Business model (funding, resources, expenses, billing)	All separate	Separate funding (may share grants), may share facility/office expenses, separate billing	Blended funding, sharing of resources, shared expenses, billing is integrated for single billing structure	Shared funding, resources, expenses, and billing
Population being targeted	Patients for which a referral or consultation is placed	Patients for which a referral or consultation is placed, shared patients	Subgroup of the larger population, either specific patients or specific conditions	Entire clinic population, including those not seen by behavioral health clinician and those without significant behavioral issues

Fully Integrated/Collaborative

Fully integrated models consider behavioral health consultants a member of the pediatric primary care practice. In a fully integrated, collaborative IBH model, the behavioral health consultant is available and consulted during all regularly scheduled pediatric office visits.[13,16] In integrated care, instead of having two separate treatment plans (one with medical elements and one with behavioral elements) there is a unified treatment plan that includes the pediatric care and behavioral management plans.[13,16] Integrated model does not necessarily function to replace more extensive regular behavioral health care evaluation and management of children and adolescents. Rather, it functions to augment, or complement, the timely delivery of behavioral health care more efficiently and effectively in the pediatric practice setting.[13,16]

Primary Care Behavioral Health

Reiter and colleagues[12] described primary care behavioral health (PCBH) as "a team based primary care approach to managing behavioral health problems and biopsychosocially influenced health conditions." The main goal of the PCBH model is to work collaboratively with the primary medical care team in increasing the level of effectiveness of overall care delivery in the evaluation and management of behavioral health concerns seen in the primary care setting.[12] As an integral member of the primary medical care team, the behavioral health consultant is available to participate in the care of all patients seen in the practice. The behavioral health consultant participates in the care of all patients as a routine practice, and provides brief office assessments and interventions as indicated, in an efficient manner. Follow-up visits are scheduled, if indicated, for more extensive behavioral evaluation and treatment. The behavioral health consultant is embedded within the medical practice in terms of shared location and resources.

Although the PCBH and fully integrated behavioral health care models are similar in principle, they differ in what patient population is served.[3,12,16] Many fully integrated behavioral health care programs focus on improving individual patient care outcomes because these programs often target either specific patients or specific conditions. However, the main focus of the PCBH approach is to improve care of the entire practice population.[12] PCBH aims to improve population heath by strengthening primary care in general by improved access to PCP; improved access to preventive care; improved PCP comfort and skill in working with biopsychosocial issues; and by providing brief, low-intensity interventions to large numbers of patients.[13]

Hybrid Approach

Different IBH models individually may or may not best serve the needs of the practice, in which case a combination or hybrid approach would be a preferred approach. The specific needs of the medical practice and the patient population it serves are the key determinants of the most preferred IBH model for that practice (eg, collaborative model providing anxiety intervention and coordinated care with psychiatry).[15] Hybrid models highlight the diverse set of services provided by IBH and that IBH models should not be viewed as one-size-fits-all.[15]

The delivery of medical care by an interprofessional team that includes behavioral health clinicians is different than a typical primary care. In an IBH model, each team member brings with him or her a unique set of professional competencies. Each team member must acknowledge and respect the expertise of different disciplines. A clear understanding of one's role on the team and effective communication are essential.

The delivery of IBH requires a change in practice operational workflows and a cultural adaptation by the administrative and professional staff to working together in a coordinated manner. Systemic or practice level characteristics are as important as professional competencies in effective implementation of an IBH model.

SUMMARY

IBH represents a cost-effective way for pediatricians to help their patients receive necessary behavioral and mental health care without requiring the physician to devote substantially more time to provide this care in a quality manner.

CLINICS CARE POINTS

- Although there are several different models of integrated behavioral health care, they all share three basic characteristics: coordination of care, continuity of care, and comprehensive care.
- Integrated behavioral health care should not be viewed as one-size-fits-all; the model of integrated behavioral health care that a practice chooses to adopt should be based on the specific needs of the practice and the patients that the practice serves.

DISCLOSURE

The authors have nothing to disclose.

REFERENCES

1. World Health Organization and Calouste Gulbenkian Foundation. Social determinants of mental health. Geneva: World Health Organization; 2014.
2. Kessler RC, Chiu WT, Demler O, et al. Prevalence, severity, and comorbidity of 12-month DSM-IV disorders in the National Comorbidity Survey Replication [published correction appears in Arch Gen Psychiatry. 2005 Jul;62(7):709. Merikangas, Kathleen R [added]]. Arch Gen Psychiatry 2005;62(6):617–27.
3. Integrated care. Bethesda (MD): National Institute of Mental Health; 2017. Available at: https://www.nimh.nih.gov/health/topics/integrated-care/index.shtml. Accessed May 24, 2020.
4. De Hert M, Correll CU, Bobes J, et al. Physical illness in patients with severe mental disorders. I. Prevalence, impact of medications and disparities in health care. World Psychiatry 2011;10(1):52–77.
5. White KL, Williams TF, Greenberg BG. The ecology of medical care. N Engl J Med 1961;265:885–92.
6. World Health Organization, United Nations Children's Fund. Primary health care: report of the international conference on primary health care. Geneva: World Health Organization; 1978.
7. Kovner A, Knickman J, Jonas S. Jonas & Kovner's health care delivery in the United States. Tenth Edition. New York: Springer Pub; 2011. p. 318–20.
8. Starfield B, Shi L, Macinko J. Contribution of primary care to health systems and health. Milbank Q 2005;83(3):457–502.
9. Committee on Integrating Primary Care and Public Health; Board on Population Health and Public Health Practice, Institute of Medicine. Primary care and public health: exploring integration to improve population health. Washington, DC: National Academies Press (US); 2012.

10. Donaldson M, Lohr K, Vanselow N, et al. Primary care: America's health in a new era. Washington DC: National Academies Press; 1996.
11. Goroll A, Mulley A. Primary care medicine. Seventh Edition. Philadelphia: Wolters Kluwer Health; 2014.
12. Reiter JT, Dobmeyer AC, Hunter CL. The Primary Care Behavioral Health (PCBH) model: an overview and operational definition. J Clin Psychol Med Settings 2018; 25(2):109–26.
13. Peek CJ, The National Integration Academy Council. Lexicon for behavioral health and primary care integration: concepts and definitions developed by expert consensus. AHRQ Publication No.13-IP001-EF. Rockville (MD): Agency for Healthcare Research and Quality; 2013. Available at: http://integrationacademy.ahrq.gov/sites/default/files/Lexicon.pdf.
14. Soares N, Apple RW, Kanungo S. The role of integrated behavioral health in caring for patients with metabolic disorders. Ann Transl Med 2018;6(24):478.
15. Blount A. Integrated primary care: organizing the evidence. Fam Syst Health 2003;21(2):121–33.
16. Njoroge WF, Hostutler CA, Schwartz BS, et al. Integrated behavioral health in pediatric primary care. Curr Psychiatry Rep 2016;18(12):106.

Integrated Behavioral Health Care
Reflections of the Past

Donald E. Greydanus, MD, DrHC (Athens)[a],*, Roger W. Apple, PhD[b],
Summer S. Chahin, MA[c]

KEYWORDS

- History of medicine • Behavioral health • Integrated care

KEY POINTS

- Development of integrated behavioral health is part of the quest of human beings over the eons for optimal health.
- Modern medicine owes much to the thinking and discoveries of ancient Egyptian and Greco-Roman clinicians.
- Integrated behavioral health owes much to the pioneering work of University of Rochester (NY) pediatrician, Robert J. Haggerty (1925–2018) with his emphasis on Behavioral Pediatrics.

INTRODUCTION

An analysis of almost any scientific problem leads automatically to a study of its history.[1]

Only by this historical route can many problems in medicine be approached profitably.
—*Sir William Osler: 1849–1919.*

Understanding the causes and cures for illness has been a major quest of human beings over the more than 200,000 years of the existence of *Homo sapiens* who emerged out of millions of years of previous evolutionary existence.[1,2] It is not known what humans knew about the potential interplay of physiology and psychology in

[a] Western Michigan University Homer Stryker M.D. School of Medicine, 1000 Oakland Drive, Kalamazoo, MI 49008, USA; [b] Division of Pediatric Psychology, Western Michigan University Homer Stryker M.D. School of Medicine, Autism Clinic, 1000 Oakland Drive, Kalamazoo, MI 49008, USA; [c] Division of Pediatric Psychology, Western Michigan University, Western Michigan University Homer Stryker M.D. School of Medicine, 1000 Oakland Drive, Kalamazoo, MI 49008, USA
* Corresponding author.
E-mail address: Donald.greydanus@med.wmich.edu

Pediatr Clin N Am 68 (2021) 519–531
https://doi.org/10.1016/j.pcl.2021.02.008
0031-3955/21/© 2021 Elsevier Inc. All rights reserved.

health until after the emergence of Sumerian clay tablets in 3500 BC that emerged from earlier Neolithic symbols or signs.[3]

Ancient Mesopotamia

Initially, emphasis was on understanding medical illness in the ancient Mesopotamia (3100–332 BC) that included Sumer and the Akkadian, Babylonian, and Assyrian empires in modern-day Iraq. Interpretation of all health was based on principles of local religion, superstition, and observation. The Code of Hammurabi is the classic Babylonian code of law dating to 1754 BC and included laws for healers to follow that included sometimes harsh punishment for failing to heal.

In the Assyro-Babylonian religions, health was attributed to having a protective or guardian angel (divine spirit) that could be replaced by evil demons or spirits if the person committed acts that angered the ruling gods.[4] The indwelling of evil demons ("witches") would lead to poor health and premature death.

Symptomatology of what was later called mental illness was attributed to presence and actions of local or foreign witches; such features apparently suggested what would later be called psychosis, anxiety, kleptomania, conduct disorder, and others.[4,5] Management would involve various recommendations based on magic and superstition. Sumerian scholars, as now, thought of the heart in philosophic terms as seen by this poem from Sumer:

It is not the heart which leads to enmity; It is the tongue which leads to enmity.

A hating heart destroys the home....[3]

Ancient Egyptian Medicine

My heart, my mother; my heart, my mother! My heart whereby I came into being!
— The Prayer of Ani, Book of the Death[6]

Current understanding of ancient Egyptian medicine (3300–525 BC) comes from information found in the Ebers Papyrus, a document dating back to 1536 BC during the time of Amenophis I (second Egyptian King of the 18th Dynasty); it was discovered by the German Egyptologist, Georg Ebers (1837–1898).[6,7] The Edwin Smith Papyrus is named for an American collector and dealer, Edwin Smith (1822–1906), who found this text in 1862 near Luxor, Egypt, which is the oldest known document of surgery.[7]

Ancient Egyptian physicians were also concerned with evil demons causing disease, and the Ebers Papyrus mentions various chants (incantations) and bad-smelling products to apply to persons to discourage the presence of various demons with abilities to cause illnesses; hundreds of prescriptions were also found in this document, and these medications were from various sources—vegetable, mineral, and animal.[8–10]

One area of the papyrus called "Book of the Hearts" deals with mental illness that included such conditions as dementia, psychosis, and depression; problems with the heart led to anger and depression. In ancient Egyptian thought, the heart was identified as the center of emotion, thought, and memory. However, continuing then as now was the daunting influence of mantics, magic, mysticism, haruspex, and religion.

Ancient Greek Medicine

The first known Greek school of medicine was established in Cnidus in 700 BC and one of its first famous medical leaders was Alcmaeon of Croton (born around 510 BC) who noted that one must observe one's patients to understand principles of disease.[11] Separating scientific principles from magic and religion remained a daunting task then and perhaps now.

A major leader in this direction was not a physician but a historian, Thucydides (460–400 BC) of Athens, Greece. Thucydides wrote the famous work, *History of the Peloponnesian War*, that provided a historical account of the fifth century BC between Athens and Sparta. In this classic account, he included events that were based on verifiable data and not myths based on effects of the Greek gods. This father of scientific history began the slow but steady march toward scientific understanding of science that included medicine.[11]

Hippocrates of Kos (460–370 BC) is called the father of Western medicine, as he sought to look at medicine more from a scientific viewpoint than one based on religion, magic, and superstition. He wrote about "hysteria" in women and also epilepsy that was called the "sacred" disease.[11] His views were recorded by his students in the Corpus Hippocraticum. Treatment of disorders including behavioral problems remained in its infancy. Aristotle (384–322 BC) was a famous student of the great Greek philosopher, Plato (427–347 BC). Aristotle, also a physician, noted that "...*the physician does not cure man, except in an incidental sense.*"

Medicine remained rooted in the classic theory of humorism or the balance of the 4 classic humors: black bile, yellow bile, phlegm, and blood. Such a view persisted into the sixteenth century in Europe. Its struggle to look at all disease objectively and scientifically remained. One of the great philosophers of all time, Socrates (470–399 BC), offered some hope in this regard as well as some advice for future clinicians:

Medicine does not consider the interests of medicine, but the interests of the patient... No physician, insofar as he is a physician, considers his own good in what he practices, but the good of his patient.
— Socrates in Plato's Republic

Ancient Roman Medicine: Galen

He cures most successfully in whom the people have the greatest confidence (Galen, 180 CE)

Claudius Galen (130–200 AD) is the famous Greek physician from Pergamum (Turkey) who was the physician to the gladiators and others in Rome, Italy. He stimulated the views of Hippocrates and is called the Roman father of medicine. He distinguished between sematic and functional disorders and concluded that neurologic illness represented a physical basis for behavioral problems. He also continued the Hippocratic view that excessive sexual behavior was harmful to youth.[12] He linked masturbation in youth as causative in several unexplained disorders—such as depression, epilepsy, acne, and others. Galen warned his society about the evils of masturbation[12]:

Watch carefully over this young man, leave him along neither night or day; at least sleep in his chamber. When he has contracted his fatal habit, the most fatal to which a young man can be subject, he will care its painful effects to the tomb— his mind and body will always be enervated.

Post-Dark Ages Progress in Pediatrics

The influence of Galen was profound and lasted well into the Renaissance era (fourteenth century into the sixteenth century in Europe) and even to the present day.[13] Dealing with behavioral versus medical problems in children and adolescents was not part of this post-Galenic legacy, as intellectual energy tended to be on adult problems and not those of children.[14]

The fall of Rome in 476 AD led to the Dark Ages (476–800 AD) with loss of vital medical information that was fortunately saved and advanced by brilliant clinicians in the Middle East. For example, the famous Persian physician Rhazes (Muhammad ibn Zakariya Razi [865–925 AD]) advanced knowledge about children's diseases with his book on pediatrics.[11,14]

The West slowly awoke from its post-Dark ages slumber, and a textbook dealing with children was published in 1050 CE by Trotula Platearius of Salerno, Italy; it was called *De Mylierum Passionibus*.[11] An important textbook on children was published by Englishman Thomas Phaer (1510–1560) in 1544 called *The Boke of Chyldren*; the author was a physician as well as a lawyer, and he made important distinctions between stages of children versus adulthood that set the stage for studies of both mental and physical health over the centuries to follow.[11,14–16]

The rights of children were emphasized by the brilliant and influential John Locke (1632–1704); this English physician and philosopher set the stage for further research into disorders of children.[17] In the eighteenth century the Swedish physician, Nils Rosén von Rosenstein (1706–1773), wrote a textbook on pediatrics called *The diseases of children and their remedies*.[18–21] In his book, this often called "father of modern pediatrics" contrasted the nerves of children versus adults: *"the nerves of children were very irritable and much more softened, and also covered with very thin membranes.[14,21]"*

Children and Nineteenth Century Progress

The beginning of the nineteenth century witnessed the start of the great children's hospital in Paris—L'Hôpital des Enfants-Malades (1802), and the middle of the nineteenth century ushered in the great London children's hospital—the Great Ormond Street Children's Hospital in 1852.[22] As medical disorders of children were being studied, knowledge of behavioral issues slowly emerged. For example, the famous German writer/illustrator and physician, Heinrich Hoffmann (1809–1894), wrote an 1846 story about a boy with probable attention-deficit/hyperactivity disorder (ADHD): Die Geschichte vom Zappel-Philipp (The story of fidgety Philip); this description was part of a book about children with the title "Struwwelpeter" (Slovenly Peter; Straw Peter).[23]

John Milton Scudder (1829–1894) was an American physician who published a book in 1869 dealing with children's diseases; in his work he noted that children were capable of *"receiving mental impressions and being pleasurably or painfully impressed by them…(children) are more impressionable than the adult.[24]"* He advocated study of children because *"there are sufficient differences in the action of remedies upon the adult and the child to demand a careful study of the subject"* (ie, the child).[24]

The influential German neurologist and psychiatrist, Wilhelm Griesinger (1817–1868), wrote in 1867 that mental illness or insanity could occur in children using English terms such as "melancholia" and "mania."[22,25] The English geologist and naturalist of enormous fame, Charles Robert Darwin (1809–1882), published his opus magnus, *On the Origin of the Species*, in 1859; in 1872 Darwin published *Expression of the Emotions in Man and Animals* that provided observations on human psychology evolution based, in part, on consultations with nineteenth century mental health experts such as Sir James Crichton-Browne (1840–1938).[26–29]

The father of psychoanalysis, Austrian neurologist and psychiatrist, Sigmund Freud (1856–1939), emphasized the importance of working with people in a counseling setting to help them work through their mental health problems.[30–32] However, the beginning of official recognition of psychiatric disorders in children and adolescents is often attributed to the insightful German (Weimar) psychiatrist, Hermann Emminghaus (1845–1904); his 1887 monumental publication, *Die psychischen Störungen des Kindesalters* (*Psychic Disturbances in Childhood*) was the start of pediatric psychiatry in Europe.[22,33–36] Mental health issues in pediatric patients, such as depression and suicidal behavior, were acknowledged and management principles developed.[22,35]

A French physician, Charles Louis Maxime Durand-Fardel (1815–1889), stimulated interest in pediatric mental health by writing that children can commit suicide and that this pediatric phenomenon worsened with puberty.[22] The English physician, Daniel Hack Tuke (1827–1895), noted in 1892 that what was called "uncomplicated insanity" could, in unusual circumstances, occur in adolescents, typically because adolescence was ending.[22,37]

Mental illness was called "insanity," and means of management were debated by various clinicians. Inpatient treatment was seen in the development of various sanitariums (sanatoriums) such as the famous "Jugendsanatorium" school on Sophienhöhe (near Jena, Germany) that was started in 1892 by the German educator Johannes Trüper (1855–1921); he also was a codeveloper of an important German journal dealing with pediatric mental illness called *Die Kinderfehler* ("Children's Mistakes").[22,38]

Inpatient management of pediatric mental illnesses was also seen with the famous British psychiatrist, Henry Maudsley (1835–1918); there was his 1895 textbook and the development of a psychiatric hospital in 1923 called the Maudsley Hospital in London that provided an area for children to be treated.[22,39,40] Another concept of dealing with mentally ill youth was seen in attempts to deal with juvenile delinquents, as seen with the development of Juvenile Courts including the first Juvenile Court in Chicago, Illinois in 1899.[41,42]

Children and Twentieth Century Progress

Georg Theodor Ziehen (1862–1950) was a German psychiatrist who worked at the famous Sophienhöhe and published his influential book, *Mental Diseases in Childhood*, in the early part of the twentieth century.[43] In 1904 the famous American psychologist, G. Stanley Hall (1844–1924), published his magnus opus (*Adolescence: Its Psychology and its Relationship to Physiology, Anthropology, Sociology, Sex, Crime, Religion, and Education*) that develop cardinal concepts of adolescent development.[44]

Child psychiatry continued to advance with an important 1910 textbook in this field by German psychiatrist, Wilhelm Stromayer (1874–1936); also, there was the post-World War II establishment of an inpatient pediatric psychiatric unit by Polish/German psychiatrist, Rudolf Lemke (1906–1957), that was separate from the adult ward.[45,46]

As inpatient treatment of children and youth with mental health issues was being developed, the movement toward *outpatient therapy* and a *team-based approach* took shape in the twentieth century. A key person in this regard was American neurologist/psychiatrist William Healy (1869–1963); he was the first director of the IJR (Institute for Juvenile Research) and established the first child guidance clinic in the United States—stimulating the child guidance clinic movement in the United States and beyond in the twentieth century as well as the twenty-first century.[22,47–49]

Therapy for children and adolescents was greatly improved with improvements in pediatric intelligence testing that occurred in the twentieth century; this was seen with research by the French psychologist Alfred Binet (1857–1911), Italian psychologist Sante De Sanctis (1862–1935), Romanian-American psychologist Lewis Madison Terman (1877–1956), and the American psychologist David Wechsler (1896–1981).[50–54]

The *Wechsler-Bellevue Intelligence Scale* for adults was published in 1939, and the *Wechsler Intelligence Scale for Children* (WISC) was published in 1949.[22]

Other icons of pediatric mental health arose in the twentieth century, some of whom continued their work into the twenty-first century. These included Swiss psychiatrist Moritz Tramer (1882–1963), American behaviorist/psychologist BF Skinner (Burrhus Frederic Skinner; 1904–1990), Austrian-American psychiatrist Leo Kanner MD (1894–1981), and American child psychiatrist Leon Eisenberg (1922–2009).[22,55–62] An icon of child psychiatry and psychology that has crossed over from the twentieth to the twenty-first century is English psychologist, Sir Michael Rutter, who was born in 1933 and knighted in 1992; he is called the father of child psychology.[63–66]

These icons have enlarged our understanding of childhood psychiatry/behavioral problems that include ADHD, autism spectrum disorders, depression, anxiety disorders, and many others. A summary of current understanding of adult and pediatric psychiatric disorders is found in the 2013 publication of the American Psychiatric Association's *Diagnostic and Statistical Manual (DSM-5) of Mental Disorders*—a publication that began in the middle of the twentieth century based on research from the nineteenth and early twentieth century.[11,14,22,66,67]

Management of these conditions in children and adolescents improved with the growth of pediatric psychopharmacology. This field began in the 1930s with the use of such mental health medications as barbiturates, antihistamines, and psychostimulants.[68,69] A racemic combination of levoamphetamine and dextroamphetamine (Benzedrine) was used in the 1930s for what is now called ADHD, and methylphenidate was introduced for this condition in 1959.[70] In the early 1900s, the father of British Pediatrics, Sir George Frederic Still (1868–1941), noted some of these youth had a "*...moral defect without general impairment of intellect.*[71]"

Lithium, antidepressant medications, and benzodiazepines were available to adults before 1965, and research later in the twentieth and now twenty-first century have led to the *pediatric* use of selective serotonin reuptake inhibitors, atypical antipsychotics, and others.[22,72,73] The Multimodal Treatment Study of Children with ADHD (MTA) has refined the understanding of benefits of methylphenidate with and without therapy.[74]

Despite such progress in understanding and managing mental illness in pediatric persons, there remains more to learn about helping these individuals in the outpatient setting. A survey of 10,123 youth aged 13 to 18 years of age in the United States and published in 2010 noted that 22% had a mental health disorder with severe impairment.[75] Anxiety disorders were the most common disorder at 31.9%; then there were behavioral disorders at 19.1%, mood disorders at 14.3%, and substance use disorders at 11.4%.[75] The mean onset of anxiety disorders was 6 years; 11 years for behavioral disorders, 13 years for mood disorders, and 15 years for substance use disorders.[75]

Integrated Behavioral Health Care

He cures most successfully in whom the people have the greatest confidence
—*Galen*[11]

Galen of Pergamos (130–200 AD) led the groundwork for the development of integrated behavioral health care that would take root 2 millennia later; his comment about confidence in one's health care provider rings true today.

Indeed, the search has been to understand the basis for disease and the best way to manage it. The past centuries of health care have laid the foundation for the importance of primary care medicine and encouraging confidence in the person's doctor and allowing choice of this health care provider when possible.[76–82]

The concept of "integrative medicine" has been attributed to the Renaissance Swiss physician, Paracelsus (Philippus Aureolus Theophrastus Bombastus von Hohenheim; 1493–1541); this astrologer and alchemist advocated for a multilayered, integrative approach to health care.[83] This included the need for observation in medicine—a concept also championed by Hippocrates.[11] The issue of various forms of integrating medicine gained more and more momentum from the mid-twentieth century to the present; gradually the importance of behavioral medicine (including liaison psychiatry/psychology) in management of disease was also recognized during this time.[84–90]

Behavioral Pediatrics

Robert J. Haggerty MD (1925–2018), an icon of pediatrics in the twentieth century from the University of Rochester School of Medicine (Rochester, New York), noted that the term, *behavioral pediatrics*, was used in the early 1970s at the University of Rochester to distinguish a program dealing with emotional problems in pediatric patients based in a pediatrics program versus a psychiatry program.[91] He noted that psychologists and psychiatrists were consulting on pediatric patients in the pediatrics department, and it was based on a program that had been initiated by Stanford Friedman MD at the University of Maryland (Baltimore, Maryland).[91,92] Dr Stanford Friedman defined behavioral pediatrics as "an area within pediatrics which focuses on the psychological, social, and learning problems of children and adolescents."[92]

As the twentieth century closed, more interest and information developed on the importance of behavioral pediatrics and its integration into primary care.[93–95] Mental health specialists (ie, psychiatrists, psychologists, and others) in this early part of the twenty-first century are working in primary care clinics (ie, family practice, pediatrics, and others) in various professional relationships that include colocated and non-colocated mental health settings.[96–102] A variety of therapies can be offered in behavioral and primary psychiatric programs, including psychosocial therapies for those with depression, anxiety disorders, substance abuse disorder, and others.[98–105] Issues of reimbursement continue to be studied in the fiscal concerns of twenty-first century medicine.[106–108]

SUMMARY

Those having torches will pass them on to others.

—Plato, The Republic[11]

Humans have long sought to be provided with optimal health care and the research continues in the twenty-first century. In the spirit of Galen from 19 centuries ago, empowering the patient's physician remains an important approach in health care. There is an emphasis on primary care and integration of behavioral consultation services in primary care.[109–112] It remains a work in progress with help from the past and realistic hope for the future.[113–115]

The philosophers thought it proper to put not 1 but 2 mottoes on the Temple at Delphi: one, the better remembered, was "Know Thyself": but the second, equally imperative, enjoined "Nothing in Excess."[116]

CLINICS CARE POINTS

- Integrated primary care and behavioral consultation services seek to improve behavioral health in pediatric persons.

- Medical illness is linked with mental illness and mental health in human beings.
- Periodically an enlightened clinical scholar provides insight into the mysteries of human health.
- Understanding of what humans have believed about health and why these beliefs developed can point the way to future insights into integrated behavioral health linked with medical illness.

DISCLOSURE

The authors do not have any conflict of interest.

REFERENCES

1. Magner LN. A history of the life sciences. third edition. New York: Marcel Dekker; 2002.
2. Patterson N, Richter DJ, Gnerre S, et al. Genetic evidence for complex speciation of humans and chimpanzees. Nature 2006;441(7097):1103–8.
3. Kramer SN. The sumerians. Chicago: The University of Chicago Press; 1963. p. 225–6.
4. Paulissian R. Medicine in ancient Assyria and Babylonia. J Assyr Acad Stud 1991;5(1):2–51.
5. Kinnier-Wilson JV. An introduction to Babylonian psychiatry. Assyriological studies. Chicago, Illinois: Oriental Institute of the University of Chicago; 1965. p. 289–98.
6. Taylor John H, editor. Ancient Egyptian book of the dead: journey through the afterlife. London, England: British Museum Press; 2010. p. 54.
7. Hallmann-Mikolajczak A. Ebers Papyrus. The book of the medical knowledge of the 16th century B.C. Egyptians. Arch Hist Filoz Med 2004;67(1):5–14 [In Polish].
8. Available at: http://www.crystalinks.com/egyptmedicine.html. Accessed March 20, 2021.
9. Grollman AP. Alternative medicine: The importance of evidence in medicine an medical evidence. Foreward: Is there wheat among the chaff? Acad Med 2001; 76(3):221–3.
10. Porter R. The greatest benefit to mankind: a medical history of humanity. New York: WW Norton; 1998.
11. Greydanus DE, Merrick J. Medical history, some perspectives. NY: Nova Biomedical; 2016. p. 216.
12. Greydanus DE, Geller B. Masturbation: historical perspectives. N Y State Med 1980;80:1892–6.
13. Shoja MM, Tubbs RS, Ghabili K, et al. The Roman Empire legacy of Galen (129-200 AD). Childs Nerv Syst 2015;31(1):1–5.
14. Greydanus DE, Patel DR, Feucht C. Preface. Pediatric and adolescent psychopharmacology: the past, the present, and the future. Pediatr Clin North Am 2011;58(1):xv–xxiv.
15. Brian VA. Thomas Phaier. First author in English on children's diseases. Nurs Mirror Midwives J 1977;144(8):59–60.
16. Bloch H. Thomas Phaer, MD (1510-1560): father of English pediatrics. South Med J 1990;83(6):672–4.

17. Williams AN. Physician, philosopher, and paediatrician: John Locke's practice of child health care. Arch Dis Child 2006;91(1):85–9.
18. Sjögren I. Nils Rosén von Rosenstein—the father of paediatrics. Ups J Med Sci 2006;111(1):3–16.
19. Lind J. Nils Rosen Von Rosenstein. Swedish pioneer in pediatrics, on the occasion of the 2D centenary of the publication of his book: "Treatice on Pediatrics". Presse Med 1964;72:2073–4 [In French].
20. Segerstedt TT. Nils Ros'en von Rosenstein and his textbook on Paediatrics. Acta Paediatr Suppl 1964;156(Suppl):7–8.
21. Hjarne U. The life and work of Nils Rosen von Rosenstein. Nord Med 1957; 57(21):740–3 [In Swedish].
22. Greydanus DE, Merrick J. Pediatric psychopharmacology: perspectives of history. In: Greydanus DE, Calles JL, Patel DR, et al, editors. Clinical aspects of psychopharmacology in childhood and adolescence. Second Edition. NY: Nova Biomedical; 2017. p. 3–32.
23. Thome J, Jacobs KA. Attention deficit hyperactivity disorder (ADHD) in a 19th century children's book. Eur Psychiatry 2004;19(5):303–6.
24. Scudder JM. The eclectic practice of diseases of children. Cincinnati, Ohio: American Publishing Co; 1869. p. 19.
25. Dietze HJ, Voegele GE. Wilhelm Griesinger's contributions to dynamic psychiatry. Dis Nerv Syst 1965;26(9):579–82.
26. Delisle RG. Evolution in a fully constituted world: Charles Darwin's debts towards a static world in the Origin of Species (1859). Endeavour 2014;38(3 4):197–210.
27. Burghardt GM. Darwin's legacy to comparative psychology and ethology. Am Psychol 2009;64(2):102–11.
28. Jacyna S. The most important of all the organs: Darwn on the brain. Brain 2009; 132(Pt 12):3481–7.
29. Pearn AM. 'This excellent observer...': the correspondence between Charles Darwin and James Crichton-Browne, 1969-75. Hist Psychiatry 2010;21(82 Pt 2):160–75.
30. Gedo JE. The enduring scientific contributions of Sigmund Freud. Perspect Biol Med 2002;45(2):200–11.
31. Tan SY, Takeyesu A. Sigmund Freud (1856-1939): father of psychoanalysis. Singapore Med J 2011;52(5):322–3.
32. Freud S. Critical introduction to neuropathology (1885-1887). Sigmund Freud. Published by Katja Guenther, Gerhard Fichtner and Albrecht Hirschmüller. Luzif Amor 2012;25(49):33–82 [In German].
33. Nissen G. Hermann Emminghaus. Founder of scientific child and adolescent psychiatry. Z Kinder Jugendpsychiatr 1986;14(1):81–7.
34. Harms E. At the cradle of child psyciatry. Hermann Emminghaus' Psychische Stoerungen des Kindesalters (1887). Am J Orthopsychiatry 1960;30:186–90.
35. Lobert W. Psychodynamic aspects of depression and suicidal behavior in childhood and adolescence—with reference to the monograph by Hermann Emminghaus 1887. Psychiatr Neurol Med Psychol (Leipz) 1987;39(11):686–92 [In German].
36. Daute KH, Lobert W. Hermann Emminghaus. 100 years of the psychopathology of childhood and adolescence. Psychiatr Neurol Med Psychol (Leipz) 1987; 39(11):682–5 [In German].
37. No authors listed. Daniel Hack Tuke. Br J Psychiatry 1995;166(3):403–5.

38. Gerhard UJ, Schönberg A, Blanz B, et al. Mediator between child and adolescent psychiatry and pedagogy. Z Kinder Jugendpsychiatr Psychother 2008; 36(1):55–63 [In German].
39. Johnston W, Williams JF. Henery Fitzgerald Maudsley. Med J Aust 1962;49(2): 520–2.
40. The Maudsley Hospital. Opening Ceremony. Br Med J 1923;1(3240):196.
41. Roberts AR, Brownell P. A century of forensic social work: bridging the past to the present. Soc Work 1999;44(4):359–69.
42. Bradley K. Juvenile delinquency, the juvenile courts, and the settlement movement 1908-1950: Basil Henriques and Toynbee Hall. 20 Century Br Hist 2008; 19(2):133–55.
43. Gerhard UJ, Blanz B. Theodor Ziehen as child and adolescent psychiatrist. A belated commemoration on the 50th anniversary of his death. Z Kinder Jugendpsychiatr Psychother 2002;30(2):127–33 [In German].
44. Stanley Hall: adolescence: its psychology and its relationship to physiology, Anthropology, Sociology, Sex, Crime, religion, and education. NY: D. Appleton and Co; 1904.
45. Frings M. Wilhelm Strohmayer (1874-1936). Nervenartz 2004;75(7):694–5 [In German].
46. Gerhard UJ, Gerhard C, Blanz B. Rudolf Lemke's contribution to the development of child neuropsychiatry in Jena, Germany. Nervenartz 2007;78(6): 706–12 [In German].
47. Snodgrass J. William Healy (1869-1963): pioneer child psychiatrist and criminologist. J Hist Behav Sci 1984;20(4):332–9.
48. Gardner GE. William Healy. 1869-1963. J Am Acad Child Psychiatry 1972; 11(1):1–29.
49. Mundie GS. Child guidance clinics. Can Med Assoc J 1924;14(6):508–11.
50. Silverman HL, Krenzel K. Alfred Binet: prolific pioneer in psychology. Psychiatr Q Suppl 1964;38:323–35.
51. Boake C. From the Binet-Simon to the Wechsler-Bellevue: tracing the history of intelligence testing. J Clin Exp Neuropsychol 2002;24(3):383–405.
52. Cicciola E, Foschi R, Lombardo GP. Making up intelligence scales: De Sanctis's and Binet's tests, 1905 and after. Hist Psychol 2014;17(3):223–36.
53. Hilgard ER. Lewis Madision Terman: 1877-1956. Am J Psychol 1957;70(3): 472–9.
54. Wechsler D. Intellectual development and psychological maturity. Child Dev 1950;21(1):45–50.
55. Kanner L. A tribute to Moritz Trarmer. Acta Paedopsychiatr 1963;30:281–4.
56. Eliasberg WG. In memoriam: Moritz Tramer, M.D. (1882-1963). Am J Psychiatry 1964;121:103–4.
57. Keller FS. Burrhus Frederic Skinner (1904-1990). J Hist Behav Sci 1991; 27(1):3–6.
58. Eisenberg L. Leo Kanner, M.D. 1894-1981. Am Psychiatry 1981;138(8):1122–5.
59. Bender L. In memoriam. Leo Kanner MD June 13, 1894-April 4, 1981. J Am Acad Child Psychiatry 1982;21:88–9.
60. Harris J. Leon Eisengerg MD (1922-2009). J Am Acad Child Adolesc Psychiatry 2010;49(2):199–201.
61. Eisenberg L. Psychiatry and human rights: putting the good of the patient first. Actas Esp Psiquiatr 2009;37(1):1–8.
62. Eisenberg L, Belfer M. Prerequisites for global child and adolescent mental health. J Child Psychol Psychiatry 2009;50(1):26–35.

63. Kolvin I. The contribution of Michael Rutter. Br J Psychiatry 1999;174:471–5.
64. Rutter J. Psychosocial resilience and protective mechanisms. Amer J Orthopsychiatry 1987;57(3):316–31.
65. Rutter M. Autism research: lessons from the past and prospects for the future. J Autism Dev Disord 2005;35(2):241–57.
66. Musto DF. History of child psychiatry. In: Lewis M, editor. Child and adolescent psychiatry. A comprehensive text. Third Edition. Philadelphia, PA: Lippincott Williams Wilkins; 2002. p. 1448–9.
67. American Psychiatric Association. Diagnostic and statistical manual of mental disorders. Fifth Edition. Arlington, VA: American Psychiatric Association; 2013.
68. Bradley C. The behavior of children receiving benzadrine. Am J Psychiatry 1937;94:577–85.
69. Molitch M, Sullivan J. The effect of benzedrine sulfate on children taking the new Stanford achievement test. Am J Orthopsych 1937;7:519–22.
70. Knobel M, Wolman M, Mason A. Hyperkinesis and organicity in children. Arch Gen Psychiatry 1959;1(3):310–21.
71. Still GF. Some abnormal psychical conditions in children: excerpts from three lectures. J Atten Disord 2006;10:126.
72. March J, Silva S, Petrycki S. Fluoxetine, cognitive-behavioral therapy, and their combination for adolescents with depression: Treatment for Adolescents with Depression Study (TADS) randomized controlled trial. JAMA 2004;292:807–20.
73. FDA panel OKs 3 antipsychotic drugs for pediatric use, cautions against overuse. JAMA 2009;302:833–4.
74. Molina BS, Hinshaw SP, Eugene AL, et al. Adolescent substance use in the multimodal treatment study of attention-deficit/hyperactivity disorder (ADHD) (MTA) as a function of childhood ADHD, random assignment to childhood treatments, and subsequent medication. J Am Acad Child Adolesc Psychiatry 2013; 52(3):250–63.
75. Merikangas KR, He JP, Burstein M, et al. Lifetime prevalence of mental disorders in US adolescents: results from the National Comorbidity Survey Replication—Adolescent Supplement (NCS-A). J Am Acad Child Adolesc Psychiatry 2010; 49(10):980–9.
76. Roemer MI. The importance of free choice of doctor and its weight in organization of medical care. Isr J Med Sci 1974;10(1):141–57.
77. Saunders DE Jr. Education for primary health care: the importance of character training. J Med Educ 1971;46(7):613–5.
78. Schor EL. American Academy of Pediatrics Task Force on the Family. Pediatrics 2003;111(6 Pt 2):1541–71.
79. Sprague L. Fitness, knowledge, progress: assessing physician qualification. Issue Brief Natl Health Policy Forum 2006;(809):1–12.
80. Kringos DS, Boerma WG, Hutchinson A, et al. The breadth of primary care: a systematic literature review of its core dimensions. BMC Heatlh Serv Res 2010;10:65.
81. Gann B. Giving patients choice and control: health informatics on the patient journey. Yearb Med Inform 2012;7:70–3.
82. Martino SC, Grob R, Davis S, et al. Choosing doctors wisely: can assisted choice enhance patients' selection of clinicians? Med Care Res Rev 2017; 76(5):572–96.
83. Thilo-Körner DG. Health-disease: theory and practice of "integrative medicine". Praxis (Bern 1994) 1994;83(51–52):1448–54 [In German].

84. No authors listed. Administrative and integrative patterns of medicine. J Med Educ 1952;27(3–1):180–1.

85. Schwartz GE, Shapiro AP, Redmond DP, et al. Behavioral medicine approaches to hypertension: an integrative analysis of theory and research. J Behav Med 1979;2(4):311–63.

86. Natelson BH. Medicine in the '90s. Need for an integrative approach. Am J Med 1986;81(6):1048–50.

87. Newman MA. Toward an integrative model of professional practice. J Prof Nurs 1990;6(3):167–73.

88. Bourgeois M. Health psychology, medical psychology, psychosomatic medicine, and liaison psychiatry. Ann Med Psychol (Paris) 1994;152(10):674–82 [In French].

89. Fortney L, Rakel D, Rindfleisch JA, et al. Introduction to integrative primary care: the health-oriented clinic. Prim Care 2010;37(1):1–12.

90. Maizes V, Rakel D, Niemiec C. Integrative medicine, and patient-centered care. Explore (NY) 2009;5(5):277–89.

91. Haggerty RJ. Foreword: Behavioral Pediatrics, 1st Edition, 1992. In: Greydanus DE, Patel DR, Pratt HD, et al, editors. Behavioral pediatrics. Fourth Edition. NY: Nova Biomedical; 2015. p. xvii–xviii.

92. Friedman SB. Symposium on behavioral pediatrics. Pediatr Clin North Am 1975; 22:55.

93. Greydanus DE, Patel DR, Pratt HD. Behavioral Pediatrics, Part I. Pediatr Clin North Am 2003;50(4):741–961.

94. Greydanus DE, Patel DR, Pratt HD. Preface, Behavioral Pediatrics, Part II. Pediatr Clin North Am 2003;50:963–1231.

95. Greydanus DE, Pratt HD, Patel DR. Behavior Pediatrics. Prim Care Clin 2007; 34(2):177–444.

96. Jansen DEMC, Krol B, Goothoff JW, et al. Towards improving medical care for people with intellectual disability living in the community: possibilities of integrated care. J Appl Res Intellect Disabil 2006;19:214–8.

97. Kathol RG, Butler M, McAlpine DD, et al. Barriers to physical and mental condition integrated service delivery. Psychosomat Med 2010;72(6):511–8.

98. Smith GC. From consultation-liaison psychiatry to integrated care for multiple and complex needs. Aust NZ J Psychiatry 2009;43(1):1–12.

99. Auxier A, Runyan C, Mullin D, et al. Behavioral health referrals and treatment initiation rates in integrated primary care: A Collaborative Care Research Network study. Transl Behav Med 2012;2(3):337–44.

100. Williams A, Ervin. Integration of mental and behavioral health in primary care.. In: Rubin IL, Merrick J, Greydanus DE, et al, editors. Health care for people with intellectual and developmental disabilities across the Lifespan. Switzerland: Springer International Publishing; 2016. p. 1699–707, ch 133.

101. Hacker K, Goldstein J, Link D, et al. Pediatric provider processes for behavioral health screening, decision making, and referral in sites with collocated mental health services. J Dev Behav Pediatr 2013;34(9):680–7.

102. Collins C, Hewson DL, Munger R, et al. Evolving models of health integration in primary care. Available at: http://www.milbank.org/uploads/documents/10430EvolvingCare.pdf. Accessed March 20, 2021.

103. Pratt HD. Point-counterpoint: psychotherapy in the age of pharmacology. Pediatr Clin North Am 2011;58(1):1–9.

104. Kamboj MK, Tareen RS. Management of non-psychiatric medical conditions presenting with psychiatric manifestations. Pediatr Clin North Am 2011;58(1): 219–41.
105. Nazeer A, Liepman MR. Psychosocial treatments for substance use disorders. In: Greydanus DE, Kaplan G, Patel DR, et al, editors. Substance abuse in adolescents and young adults: a manual for pediatric and primary care clinicians. Boston, Berlin: De Gruyter; 2013. p. 63–83, chapter 5.
106. Kautz C, Mauch D, Smith SA. Reimbursement of mental health services in primary care settings. Rockville: Center for Mental Health Services, Substance Abuse and Mental Health Services Administration, HHS Pub No SMA-08-4324; 2008.
107. Wiseman T. Competitive long-term health insurance. J Health Econ 2018;58: 144–50.
108. Sutton M, Garfield-Birkbeck S, Martin G, et al. Economic analysis of service and delivery interventions in health care. Southampton, UK: NIHR Journals Library; 2018. Health Services and Delivery Research.
109. Rousseau C, Pontbriand A, Nadeau L, et al. Perception of inter-professional collaboration and co-location of specialists and primary care teams in youth mental health. J Can Acad Child Adolesc Psychiatry 2017;26(3):198–204.
110. Institute for Health Care Improvement: IHI 90-Day R & D Project Final Summary Report: Integrating behavioral health and primary care. Cambridge, MA: Institute for Health Care Improvement. Available at: http://www.ihi.org/resources/Pages/Publications/BehavioralHealthIntegrationIHI90DayRDProject.aspx. Accessed March 20, 2021.
111. Weeks J. Multimodal approaches in integrative health: Whole persons, whole practices, whole systems—An invitation to submit to JACM's special issue. J Altern Complement Med 2018. https://doi.org/10.1089/acm.2018.29045.jjw.
112. Golom FD, Schreck JS. The journey to interprofessional collaborative practice: Are we there yet? Pediatr Clin North Am 2018;65(1):1–12.
113. History of medicine. Br Med J 1858;1(93):852–4.
114. Rovesti M, Fioranelli M, Petrelli P, et al. Health and illness in history, science, and society. Open Access Maced J Med Sci 2018;6(1):163–5.
115. Greydanus DE, Patel DR, Pratt HD, et al. Behavioral pediatrics: dilemmas, challenges, and faith in the future. In: Behavioral pediatrics. Fourth Edition. NY: Nova Science Publisher, Inc; 2015. p. xxv–xxxiii.
116. Lewis A. Ebb and flow in social psychiatry. Yale J Biol Med 1962;35:62–83.

Need for Integrated Behavior Health Model in Primary Care

Kevin Cates, MD, MPH[a], Neelkamal Soares, MD[b],*

KEYWORDS

- Behavioral health • Integrated behavioral health • Access

KEY POINTS

- The need for behavioral health care in primary care pediatric clinics is high, whereas access is limited.
- Primary care providers attempt to provide these services to the extent possible, but they need more support to deliver this care.
- Various strategies are emerging to integrate behavior health into primary care pediatric settings; however, individual clinical settings likely require strategies to meet the unique needs of each setting.

BACKGROUND

Behavioral health concerns are highly prevalent in patients seen in primary care pediatric clinics. Approximately 17.4% of children aged 2 years to 8 years have at least 1 mental, behavioral, or developmental disorder,[1] and an additional 20% of children do not meet criteria for a diagnosed disorder but have "clinically significant impairment or problems."[2] Approximately 1 in 7 children experience a behavioral or mental health (MH) concern requiring treatment, counseling, or referral by 21 years of age.[3] The American Academy of Pediatrics (AAP) Task Force on Mental Health estimated that by the year 2020, MH care would constitute a significant part of general pediatric practice.[4]

Accurate estimation of the prevalence of pediatric behavioral and MH conditions are hampered by shifting diagnostic criteria and changes in screening tools and screening practices, as well as ever-changing cultural perceptions of behavioral and MH issues.[5] Both the AAP and the American Academy of Child and Adolescent Psychiatry endorse children needing to access MH screening and assessment; they recommend that this

[a] Harvard South Shore Psychiatry Residency, 940 Belmont Street, Psychiatry 116A7, Brockton, MA 02301, USA; [b] Western Michigan University Homer Stryker M.D. School of Medicine, 1000 Oakland Drive, Kalamazoo, MI 49008, USA
* Corresponding author.
E-mail address: neelkamal.soares@med.wmich.edu

Pediatr Clin N Am 68 (2021) 533–540
https://doi.org/10.1016/j.pcl.2021.02.009
0031-3955/21/© 2021 Elsevier Inc. All rights reserved.

pediatric.theclinics.com

occur in the child's medical home, because the primary care clinician has unique opportunities to engage children and families in MH care without stigma.[6]

Another complicating factor is the low rates of identification by pediatricians; in a study of preschool children, pediatrician evaluation of behavior had a sensitivity of 20.5% and specificity of 92.7%, compared with independent evaluations of child psychologists.[7] This is despite the fact that pediatricians endorse that they should be responsible for identifying children with several MH and behavior problems.[8] Part of the concern is the actual discussion of MH and psychosocial health at the provider visit. Studies have shown this happens more often when the presentation was hyperactivity or when a provider had greater confidence in their MH treatment skills but less often when a child demonstrated physical pain.[9] Additionally, parents with authoritarian parenting styles are less likely to have children identified with MH problems by their primary care provider (PCP).[10] Pediatricians consistently report, however, that they lack training in identification and treatment of child MH problems and lack confidence to treat children with counseling, despite mandatory training for developmental-behavioral problems during residency.[11] Additionally, lack of confidence in diagnosing and treatment with medications, inadequate reimbursement, and lack of time have been reported as barriers.[12] Physician discomfort with their ability to treat behavioral and MH issues may contribute to a reluctance to bring up these issues and confusion over the availability and utilization of support services.[13] Although PCPs manage a large proportion of psychiatric medications in children,[14] many pediatricians remain uncomfortable with prescribing psychopharmacology and may benefit from additional training and support in this area.[15]

DISCUSSION
Current Strategies

The AAP Bright Futures initiative[16] and Mental Health Toolkit[17] provide tools for the PCP to integrate MH care in the context of routine pediatric health supervision. There has been guidance for pediatricians to implement behavioral and emotional screening in practice through operational strategies, resource identification, and greater collaboration with MH specialists and systems.[18] Data from the 1995 to 2010 National Ambulatory Medical Care Surveys indicate a trend toward more robust identification of psychiatric and behavioral issues in pediatric populations. MH and behavioral diagnoses by pediatricians increased over time, from 7.78% of visits to 15.30% of visits in 1995 and 2010, respectively.[19] This increase in diagnoses outpaced similar increases in adult care settings, suggesting either an increase in presentation or an increase in identification in primary care pediatric settings.

Barriers remain as behavioral visits frequently are time-consuming, taxing all involved (the child, caregiver, and physician).[20] They also represent an opportunity cost because they yield lower reimbursement than nonbehavioral visits. Reimbursement for each minute spent with patients presenting with medical issues without behavioral concerns is 413% higher than patients presenting with behavioral concerns, and the amount of time spent with behavioral patients is approximately double the time spent with patients without behavioral concerns.[21]

Despite improved identification, there continues to be an unmet need with 80% of children under age 17 not receiving the behavioral or psychiatric care they need,[22] with unmet need rising over the previous decade through 2010.[23] Some of this unmet need is attributed to barriers to accessing qualified MH professionals. Although children in general tend to have better coverage for MH issues than adults, pediatricians were more likely than other PCPs to report not getting outpatient MH services because of shortage of providers.[24] Geography also plays a role, because most child and adolescent psychiatric services in the United States are coalesced around urban areas, with children in rural areas and areas of low socioeconomic status having significantly reduced access.[25] Even when child psychiatrists are available, the wait times to see one can be as long as 10 weeks.[26] Administrative barriers also exist; behavioral health carve-outs were supposed to lower costs and maintain or improve access to care,[27] but studies showed that they were associated with greater unmet MH care need as compared with fee-for-service models, possibly due to increased administrative complexity and a lack of a single point of accountability.[27] Working with an external provider is a typical model, and requires coordination by the PCP office (both for sharing of documentation and scheduling). Generally shared treatment plan formulations are the goal with some return to PCP for follow-up services.[28] Limitations include the barriers, described previously, and the logistical challenges working with off-site MH providers and collaborating on care infrastructure.[29]

Newer Approaches

To address some of these concerns, several strategies have been suggested to deliver pediatric behavioral health services. There have not been studies to compare 1 approach against another, and choice of models depend on the individual needs of communities (fiscal, resources, need, and barriers), clients (age, complexity, and payer mix), and providers (PCPs, specialists, and MH access). Overall, approaches can be categorized as on-site intervention (such as co-location or integrated behavioral health), consultation, and training for the PCP.[3]

On-site interventions allow the PCP to connect the child/adolescent to behavioral and MH services in the same appointment in which concerns are identified One example is Project LAUNCH (Linking Actions for Unmet Needs in Children's Health), which found that embedded, on-site behavioral services substantially increased pediatric PCP self-reported ability to screen for, assess, and provide MH services for young children with these concerns, although sustainability will require funding, infrastructure, and policy changes.[30]

Consultation between the PCP and specialist generally is focused clinical advice and recommendations by the specialist about care decisions, intervention and referral assistance.[3] Increasingly, to address limitations and access barriers, regional networks and statewide initiatives have been developed. In Massachusetts, a statewide network of child psychiatrists is available to pediatric clinicians for consultation. A study showed improvement in the clinicians self-reporting in caring for children with psychiatric concerns.[31] See **Table 1** for other examples of consultation state-wide psychiatry programs.

Other approaches focus on building broader collaborative networks to identify and promote best practices. An example is collaborative office rounds, a strategy utilizing joint communication between pediatricians and child psychiatrists in order to facilitate improved ability of PCPs to provide behavioral health care for children.[32]

Due to PCP-reported limitations in training and ability to manage psychiatric concerns, initiatives focused on training the PCP are increasing. One such intervention focused on screening for and treating adolescent depression; a 2-hour training resulted in an increase in screening for adolescent depression and suicidality from 49% to 74%, with persistent effects.[33] A Canadian study found that a similar training yielded improvements in PCP self-reported confidence and competence in treating children's MH and behavioral health issues, but was limited by physician unwillingness to participate in extended training sessions.[34]

Table 1
Examples of state remote consultation services for child behavioral health

State	Program Name	Features	Information
Alaska	Alaska Partnership Access Line	Phone-based, state-funded, no charge, partners with Help Me Grow Alaska to connect families to social work services	https://www.seattlechildrens.org/healthcare-professionals/access-services/partnership-access-line/pal-pak
Colorado	Colorado Pediatric Psychiatry Consultation & Access Program	Phone or Web-based consult for basic MH assessment; direct face-to-face assessments available for complex cases	https://www.coppcap.org
Florida	Florida Pediatric Psychiatry Hotline	Phone-based consultation regarding medication management issues	http://www.medicaidmentalhealth.org/fppHotline.cfm
Massachusetts	Massachusetts Child Psychiatry Access Program (MCPAP)	Phone-based free consultation available to PCPs, face-to-face consults available in complex cases; collaborates with Adolescent Substance Use and Addictions Program and MCPAP For Moms for pregnant and postpartum women. Regional hubs	https://www.mcpap.com/Default.aspx
Ohio	Pediatric Psychiatry Network	Provides diagnostic support, symptom management, and education services via phone or Web-based	https://ppn.mh.ohio.gov

Increasingly, new technologies play a central role in expanding MH and behavioral health care in primary care settings. This is achieved primarily through 2 formats: telepsychiatry and Internet-based interventions. Telepsychiatry is the delivery of psychiatric services via telephone or video communication, allowing a remotely located clinician to assess a patient, discuss their care, and prescribe treatment without requiring physical presence; similarly, remotely located psychiatrists may consult with pediatricians via telephone or video technologies.[35,36] This technology has been implemented in rural underserved areas, however underserved urban environments also may benefit from utilization.[37] Internet-based interventions are still in their infancy; however, one promising program, Competent Adulthood Transition with Cognitive Behavioral humanistic and Interpersonal Training (CATCH-IT) examined an internet-based behavioral program, paired with either motivational interviewing or brief advice. It proved effective in reducing depressive symptoms in adolescents[38] and was found to be engaging for adolescents over time, contributing to the program's success[39] and had sustained effects over

6 months.[40] Internet-based psychosocial interventions may prove to be effective, accessible, and affordable for adolescents but require additional study.[41]

The need for expanded access to behavioral health care for children is well documented and broadly acknowledged. Several strategies are emerging to meet this need in primary care pediatric settings, including onsite co-location and integration of behavioral health services, consultative services either in-person or via telehealth/video, the creation of collaborative networks between pediatricians and child psychiatrists, and expanded training for primary care pediatricians. Further study is required to determine the effectiveness of each intervention, alone or in combination.

SUMMARY

Although there is merit to each of the interventions briefly described, it is unlikely that any single approach will be sufficient to close the gap in children's MH and behavioral health care. The need is daunting, and the barriers to providing the comprehensive care required by so many children are substantial. Many are the opportunities, however, for pediatric clinicians to apply methods of improving both access to, and quality of, MH and behavioral health care. There are opportunities for creative and innovative approaches with applications of new technology and information-sharing networks of clinicians to advance the effort to meet the MH and behavioral health needs of children. Although it is beyond the scope of this individual article to describe these in greater detail, this overview represents the diversity of tools available to fill the clinician's toolkit. The other articles in this volume explore more deeply issues in providing behavioral health care in the pediatric primary care setting, including funding topics, incorporation of behavioral health training in postgraduate physician training, and the specific interventions employed.

CLINICS CARE POINTS

- Screening for behavioral health/emotional concerns continues to be recommended for pediatric primary care settings.
- State-wide behavioral health consultation services exist in several states and may improve the care provided in pediatric primary care settings.
- On-site behavioral health integration may increase self-efficacy of pediatricians caring for children with behavioral health concerns.
- Telehealth/video behavioral health services may be beneficial when on-site services are unavailable.

DISCLOSURE

Neither of the authors has any financial relationship to disclose in the subject matter or materials discussed in the article.

REFERENCES

1. Cree RA, Bitsko RH, Robinson LR, et al. Health care, family, and community factors associated with mental, behavioral, and developmental disorders and poverty among children aged 2–8 Years — United States, 2016. MMWR Morb Mortal Wkly Rep 2018;67(50):1377–83.

2. Committee on Psychosocial Aspects of Child and Family Health and Task Force on Mental Health. The Future of Pediatrics: Mental Health Competencies for Pediatric Primary Care. Pediatrics 2009;124(1):410–21.

3. Kolko DJ, Perrin E. The integration of behavioral health interventions in children's health care: services, science, and suggestions. J Clin Child Adolesc Psychol 2014;43(2):216–28.

4. Foy JM, American Academy of Pediatrics Task Force on Mental Health. Enhancing pediatric mental health care: report from the american academy of pediatrics task force on mental health. Introduction. Pediatrics 2010; 125(Supplement 3):S69–74.

5. Egger HL, Angold A. Common emotional and behavioral disorders in preschool children: presentation, nosology, and epidemiology. J Child Psychol Psychiatry 2006;47(3–4):313–37.

6. American Academy of Child and Adolescent Psychiatry Committee on Health Care Access and Economics Task Force on Mental Health. Improving mental health services in primary care: reducing administrative and financial barriers to access and collaboration. Pediatrics 2009;123(4):1248–51.

7. Lavigne JV, Binns HJ, Christoffel KK, et al. Behavioral and Emotional Problems Among Preschool Children in Pediatric Primary Care: Prevalence and Pediatricians' Recognition. Pediatrics 1993;91(3):649–55.

8. Talmi A, Muther EF, Margolis K, et al. The scope of behavioral health integration in a pediatric primary care setting. J Pediatr Psychol 2016;41(10):1120–32.

9. Brown JD, Wissow LS, Riley AW. Physician and patient characteristics associated with discussion of psychosocial health during pediatric primary care visits. Clin Pediatr (Phila) 2007;46(9):812–20.

10. Dempster RM, Wildman BG, Langkamp D, et al. Pediatrician identification of child behavior problems: the roles of parenting factors and cross-practice differences. J Clin Psychol Med Settings 2012;19(2):177–87.

11. Horwitz SM, Storfer-Isser A, Kerker BD, et al. Barriers to the identification and management of psychosocial problems: changes from 2004 to 2013. Acad Pediatr 2015;15(6):613–20.

12. Horwitz SM, Kelleher KJ, Stein REK, et al. Barriers to the identification and management of psychosocial issues in children and maternal depression. Pediatrics 2007;119(1):e208–18.

13. Wissow L, Anthony B, Brown J, et al. A common factors approach to improving the mental health capacity of pediatric primary care. Adm Policy Ment Health 2008;35(4):305–18.

14. Anderson LE, Chen ML, Perrin JM, et al. Outpatient Visits and Medication Prescribing for US Children With Mental Health Conditions. Pediatrics 2015;136(5): e1178–85.

15. Kerker BD. Training pediatric PCPs in mental health conditions increases prescribing. Brown Univ Child Adolesc Psychopharmacol Updat 2015;17(5):1–3.

16. Jellinek M, Patel B, Froehle M, Eds. Bright Futures in Practice: Mental Health—Volume II, Tool Kit. Available at: https://www.brightfutures.org/mentalhealth/pdf/tools.html. Accessed August 4, 2020.

17. American Academy of Pediatrics. Addressing Mental Health Concerns in Pediatrics: A Practical Resource Toolkit for Clinicians. 2nd edition. 2021. Available at: https://toolkits.solutions.aap.org/mental-health/home.

18. Weitzman C, Wegner L. Promoting optimal development: screening for behavioral and emotional problems. Pediatrics 2015;135(2):384–95.

19. Olfson M, Blanco C, Wang S, et al. National trends in the mental health care of children, adolescents, and adults by office-based physicians. JAMA Psychiatry 2014;71(1):81.

20. Cooper S, Valleley RJ, Polaha J, et al. Running out of time: physician management of behavioral health concerns in rural pediatric primary care. Pediatrics 2006;118(1):e132–8.

21. Meadows T, Valleley R, Haack MK, et al. Physician "Costs" in Providing Behavioral Health in Primary Care. Clin Pediatr (Phila) 2011;50(5):447–55.

22. Kataoka SH, Zhang L, Wells KB. Unmet need for mental health care among u.s. children: variation by ethnicity and insurance status. Am J Psychiatry 2002; 159(9):1548–55.

23. Roll JM, Kennedy J, Tran M, et al. Disparities in unmet need for mental health services in the United States, 1997–2010. Psychiatr Serv 2013;64(1):80–2.

24. Cunningham PJ. Beyond parity: primary care physicians' perspectives on access to mental health care. Health Aff 2009;28(3):w490–501.

25. Thomas CR, Holzer CE. The continuing shortage of child and adolescent psychiatrists. J Am Acad Child Adolesc Psychiatry 2006;45(9):1023–31.

26. Children's Hospital Association (CHA). Pediatric Workforce shortages persist 2017. Available at: www.childrenshospitals.org/workforceshortage. Accessed January 25, 2018.

27. Tang MH, Hill KS, Boudreau AA, et al. Medicaid managed care and the unmet need for mental health care among children with special health care needs. Health Serv Res 2007;43(3):882 900.

28. Aupont O, Doerfler L, Connor DF, et al. A collaborative care model to improve access to pediatric mental health services. Adm Policy Ment Heal Ment Heal Serv Res 2013;40(4):264–73.

29. Sheldrick RC, Neger EN, Perrin EC. Concerns about development, behavior, and learning among parents seeking pediatric care. J Dev Behav Pediatr 2012;33(2): 156–60.

30. Substance Abuse and Mental Health Services Administration. The Integration of Behavioral Health into Pediatric Primary Care Settings. 2017. Available at: https://healthysafechildren.org/sites/default/files/The-Integration-of-Behavioral-Health-into-Pediatric-Primary-Care-Settings.pdf. Accessed July 18, 2020.

31. Sarvet B, Gold J, Bostic JQ, et al. Improving access to mental health care for children: the massachusetts child psychiatry access project. Pediatrics 2010;126(6): 1191–200.

32. Fishman ME, Kessel W, Heppel DE, et al. Collaborative office rounds: continuing education in the psychosocial/developmental aspects of child health. Pediatrics 1997;99(4):e5.

33. Fallucco EM, Seago RD, Cuffe SP, et al. Primary care provider training in screening, assessment, and treatment of adolescent depression. Acad Pediatr 2015;15(3):326–32.

34. Servili C. An international perspective on youth mental health: the role of primary health care and collaborative care models. J Can Acad Child Adolesc Psychiatry 2012;21(2):127–9.

35. Hilty DM, Yellowlees PM, Cobb HC, et al. Models of telepsychiatric consultation–liaison service to rural primary care. Psychosomatics 2006;47(2):152–7.

36. Pignatiello A, Teshima J, Boydell KM, et al. Child and youth telepsychiatry in rural and remote primary care. Child Adolesc Psychiatr Clin N Am 2011;20(1):13–28.

37. Myers KM, Sulzbacher S, Melzer SM. Telepsychiatry with children and adolescents: are patients comparable to those evaluated in usual outpatient care? Telemed J E-health 2004;10(3):278–85.
38. Van Voorhees BW, Vanderplough-Booth K, Fogel J, et al. Integrative internet-based depression prevention for adolescents: a randomized clinical trial in primary care for vulnerability and protective factors. J Can Acad Child Adolesc Psychiatry 2008;17(4):184–96.
39. Van Voorhees BW, Fogel J, Reinecke MA, et al. Randomized clinical trial of an internet-based depression prevention program for adolescents (project CATCH-IT) in primary care: 12-week outcomes. J Dev Behav Pediatr 2009; 30(1):23–37.
40. Hoek W, Marko M, Fogel J, et al. Randomized controlled trial of primary care physician motivational interviewing versus brief advice to engage adolescents with an Internet-based depression prevention intervention: 6-month outcomes and predictors of improvement. Transl Res 2011;158(6):315–25.
41. Wozney L, Huguet A, Bennett K, et al. How do eHealth Programs for Adolescents With Depression Work? A Realist Review of Persuasive System Design Components in Internet-Based Psychological Therapies. J Med Internet Res 2017; 19(8):e266.

The Many Roles of Pediatric Integrated Behavioral Health Specialists

Check for updates

Skye Lu, DO[a],*, Theron O'Halloran, MD[b], Neelkamal Soares, MD[b]

KEYWORDS

- Integrative behavioral health • Chronic diseases • Mental health disorders
- Behavioral health concerns

KEY POINTS

- Delivering integrated behavioral health (IBH) in the primary care setting may aid in identifying any early concerns or difficulties in child development, environmental health, behavior/psychosocial issues, and other parental concerns.
- IBH can serve a variety of roles for the patient/family and the clinician, including anticipatory guidance, health promotion, mental health consultations, family support, and guidance to other resources.
- In chronic medical conditions, IBH can be especially crucial with developmental, behavioral, and social difficulties that are associated with these conditions and thus contribute to better care for the child.

INTRODUCTION

Tags: Integrative Behavioral Health, Primary Care Pediatrics, Multidisciplinary Approach, Patient-Centered Medical Home

The primary care pediatric setting is intended to provide continuous and comprehensive care throughout a child's life to ensure physical, social, emotional, and environmental well-being. Routinely scheduled well-child visits are ideal to assess developmental progress, environmental health, behavior/psychosocial issues, and other parental concerns.[1] Delivering integrated behavioral health (IBH) in the primary care setting may aid in identifying any early concerns or difficulties as well as provide resources and support when these issues first emerge, thus, promoting the child's well-being.[2] Specific areas in which IBH can be particularly helpful are psychiatric disorders and chronic diseases, as both these conditions often require complex care and multidisciplinary resources.

The authors have no disclosures.
[a] Yu Pediatrics, 325 Charles H Dimmock Parkway #600, Colonial Heights, VA 23834, USA;
[b] Western Michigan University Homer Stryker MD School of Medicine, 1000 Oakland Drive, Kalamazoo, MI 49008, USA
* Corresponding author.
E-mail address: Skalu57@gmail.com

It is estimated that 15% of children worldwide suffer from a chronic medical condition.[3] The probability of a psychiatric disorder is 4 times greater in children with a chronic illness,[4] and about 10% of children with a chronic disease have a comorbid psychiatric disorder.[4,5] Several studies have shown an increased risk of behavioral problems in children with chronic diseases.[6–9] These behavioral issues in turn can have a negative impact on the symptoms and management of a physical disease. A longitudinal study showed that poor physical health predicted future depression, and major depression increased risk for poor physical health.[10] In addition to disease progression, mental health disorders can also affect social and educational development and can continue to have an impact through adulthood.

DISCUSSION

Behavioral and psychological conditions can be categorized into internalizing and externalizing types: internalizing problems include anxiety, depression, social withdrawal, attention problems, and somatic symptoms, and externalizing problems include disruptive disorders, aggression, and violence.[9] Higher levels of internalizing problems have been found in children with chronic diseases in comparison to their healthy peers, whereas externalizing problems seem to be more disease specific.[9]

During childhood and adolescence, individuals acquire developmentally appropriate skills, including autonomy, identity formation, balancing social relationships, forming individual opinions, and exploring/developing sexuality.[11] Ongoing chronic illnesses place demands on these processes, often resulting in poor adaptation skills.[11] In addition, the burden of treatment regimens can impact social relationships. These factors, taken together or individually, can disrupt normal social and identity development.[11] Studies have shown that an adolescent's ability to recognize and cope with the effects of their illness while also navigating complex social relationships is the key to managing these psychiatric disruptions.[12] Thus, recognizing these emotional, behavioral, and developmental disturbances early in patients with chronic disease is essential to the long-term health management of these children.

The patient-centered medical home (PCMH)[13] is an ideal location for coordinating mental health care. IBH can serve a variety of roles for the patient/family and the clinician, including anticipatory guidance, health promotion, mental health consultations, family support, and guidance to other resources. In later discussion, the authors summarize some examples of situations wherein IBH can provide value in the setting of a PCMH.

INVOLVEMENT OF INTEGRATED BEHAVIORAL HEALTH

With the higher frequency of well-child visits in early childhood, IBH should be engaged early and often to establish a relationship with families and follow them as the child develops, regardless of the presence of a precipitating behavior concern. This provides an opportunity for early identification of concerns and guidance when problems first emerge rather than intervening after escalation, which often requires more intensive management. The IBH consultant can provide guidance ranging from developmentally appropriate activities that caregivers can do with the young child to promote social-emotional development to proactively addressing positive discipline, toilet training, sibling rivalry, and other issues that caregivers bring up. The incorporation of IBH helps caregivers normalize discussion of behavioral or emotional issues in a primary care setting and sets the stage for addressing mental health issues, which are as important as treating the child's physical illnesses.[14]

SCREENING
Tags: Behavioral Screening, Ages and Stages Questionnaire, Screening Techniques

IBH consultants can also be involved in screening at each well-child visit for behavioral or mental health disorders using broad-based standardized tools, such as the Pediatric Symptom Checklist[15] and Ages and Stages Questionnaire (ASQ:SE),[16] among others. Studies have shown that the combination of clinical impression and standardized screening questionnaires rather than clinical judgment alone is more sensitive in picking up developmental and behavioral problems.[17,18] By focusing on validated screening techniques, the clinician can compare parents' observations and concerns to standard universal data.[17] These screenings provide for an efficient way to identify behavioral and emotional problems. A study looking at the effects of ASQ:SE as a universal screening tool for behavioral or emotional problems found that positive screens with subsequent intervention by an integrated child psychologist in the clinic showed an improved rescreening score in more than half of the children.[19] These results stress the important role of IBH to aid in screening, identifying, treating, and referring these children. The IBH consultant can also hone in on specific concerns like depression and anxiety and can administer tools, such as the Child Depression Inventory[20] or Revised Children Manifest Anxiety Scale,[21] to evaluate specific concerns. These interventions set the stage for referral to more comprehensive diagnostics with a mental health provider, such as psychologist or psychiatrist. In the case of children with chronic diseases, given the high prevalence of behavioral issues and potential for significant social stressors, early involvement of IBH is recommended.

PSYCHOSOCIAL SITUATIONS FOR INTEGRATED BEHAVIORAL HEALTH
Tags: Parental Divorce, Parental Separation, Parental Loss, Family Conflict, Low Socioeconomic Status, Economic Disadvantage, Parental Support, Parental Child Interaction Therapy

Parental divorce, separation, or loss
A major social stressor for children includes parental divorce, separation, or loss. Children who experience family disruption are at increased risk for psychiatric and behavioral disorders.[22] Approximately 20% of bereaved children exhibit behavioral or emotional symptoms, and 1 in 5 children will likely develop a psychiatric disorder.[23] In addition, the prevalence of mental health disorders in children living with a single parent is twice that of children living in a 2-parent family (16% vs 8%, respectively).[4] There have been several theories posed to explain the cause of these behavioral issues, including parental absence, economic disadvantage, and increased family conflict.[24]

Parental absence
Based on the idea that a complete family dynamic is the key to nurturing a child's social development, the absence of a parent leads to A decrease in attention, support, and supervision. Disrupting the dynamic of 2 parental role models may result in inadequate learning of social skills, such as compromising, negotiating, and cooperating, all of which are necessary for future success.[24]

Economic disadvantage
Divorce or parental loss increases risk for economic disadvantage because of the loss of household income, potentially leading to decreased academic, nutritional, or psychosocial resources that negatively impact the child's well-being. In addition, parents of higher socioeconomic status are more likely to discuss mental health issues with their pediatrician,[25] suggesting that there is a significant proportion of unrecognized behavioral issues in children of low socioeconomic status. Referral to IBH can aid in

recognizing these issues and decreasing the gap of care to these underserved populations.

Family conflict

A hostile home environment has been shown to contribute to mental health issues, independent of whether it is a single parent or 2-parent family. This is demonstrated in a study that showed children in intact families with high conflict have a lower well-being than children in divorced families with low conflict.[24] Conflict is likely to cause significant stress on the parents, resulting in less attention to the child, thus decreasing parental support during the crucial period of child development. Children also frequently become involved in parental conflicts, which leadS to deterioration of parent-child relationships. The effects of family disruption can cause everlasting behavioral issues throughout adolescence and into adulthood. Parental divorce or loss has a large impact on the social and behavioral development of a child during crucial stages of life. Children may experience problems that may include anxiety, depression, violence, anger, and regression of developmental milestones.[23] Given the longitudinal and multifaceted effects of parental loss, IBH involvement can provide behavioral counseling, coping strategies, giving parental support and direction to appropriate ancillary resources.

Parental support and training

Even without chronic illness, children can have behavioral challenges that test the fortitude of their caregivers. Parents and caregivers play a significant role in the emotional, behavioral, and social development of their child; thus, providing support and counseling to the family is just as important as providing support to the individual child. One study showed a significant positive impact of family support programs on changing parent behavior and preventing or improving early childhood behavioral problems.[26] Specific interventions that proved to be most effective included increasing positive parent-child interactions, teaching the importance of parenting consistently, and the appropriate use of time out.[26] There was also a significant benefit to training sessions in which parents and children participated in interactive sessions where new behaviors could be practiced and mastered under live supervision.[26] Parent-child interaction therapy (PCIT) is a specific form of parental training that involves direct coaching sessions in which parents are observed through a one-way mirror and given direct, live communication and feedback.[27] During these sessions, parents practice consistent positive communication with their child in order to promote positive parent-child relationships, and learn to use positive reinforcement while ignoring many negative behaviors.[27] In a meta-analysis, PCIT was shown to significantly decrease externalizing behavior in children and improve overall child behavior and parental stress.[27] IBH can aid in this process by providing the necessary resources or direct parental support.

SUPPORT IN CHRONIC CONDITIONS
Tags: Chronic Conditions, Diabetes, Cancer, Chronic Pulmonary Conditions, Functional Gastrointestinal Disorders

Chronic conditions, such as diabetes, cancer, and asthma, can have wide ranging effects on both an individual's physical health and their emotional well-being. In children, management of the disease also can have an impact on education and peer relationships. Given that the PCMH is where a substantial amount of maintenance and surveillance of chronic disease occurs, these conditions (and their impacts) provide an opportunity for IBH intervention.

As of 2017, an estimated 10,000 children receive a new diagnosis of cancer each year between the ages of 0 and 14 years. Behavioral problems associated with cancer diagnosis span all age groups, including mood changes and anxiety. Changes in behavior of patients with cancer can be difficult to pinpoint to an actual cause because of the interplay of the disease process, social factors, and adverse effects of treatment. Treatment protocols themselves may lead to behavior problems, for example, corticosteroids effects can include changes to mood, sleep, and appetite along with many other medical complications.[28] Many invasive procedures during cancer treatment, such as blood draws and intravenous placement for chemotherapy, lead to children and adolescents developing anticipatory anxiety before appointments.[28]

Diabetes is one of the most common chronic diseases that affect children in the United States with approximately 16.9% of children between the ages of 2 and 19 being considered obese.[29] With childhood obesity on the increase, recent data show an increase in type II diabetes diagnoses; however, historically type I diabetes has been the most common form found within the pediatric population.[30] Regardless of type, depression and other psychiatric diagnoses are common in childhood diabetes.[31] Patients with poor glycemic control and recurrent cases of diabetic ketoacidosis are more likely to develop behavioral problems than their well-controlled glycemic peers.[31] Children can have difficulty in school and social situations, showing weaknesses in attention and executive functioning.[31] In addition, behavioral problems are associated with disease exacerbation, and therefore, may be considered to be secondary problems and not treated appropriately. Also, children who are obese and overweight experience higher levels of bullying both from and to their peers, negatively impacting self-esteem.[32] Frequent peer comments, along with medical visits for weight, nutrition, and exercise consults, also contribute to increased awareness of self-image.[33] With the development of low self-esteem, there is an increased risk of sadness, loneliness, and anxiety.[34]

Chronic pulmonary conditions, like asthma and cystic fibrosis, have a large impact on pediatric populations with a recent increase in prevalence.[35] Both diseases have variable presentations from mild symptoms with minimal disruption to severe and constant symptoms that may deter the individual from performing daily tasks. Children have been shown to miss more days of school than healthy counterparts and score lower on standardized tests.[36] Falling behind academically and struggling to catch up with course material can result in behavioral issues from stress.[37]

Functional gastrointestinal (GI) disorders, such as chronic constipation, irritable bowel syndrome, and functional dyspepsia, make up around 40% of all GI conditions and have prolonged effects.[38] Depression, anxiety, and panic disorders are commonly found with patients with functional GI disorder.[39] For children, there is a correlation between the length of time that their abdominal symptoms are present and the severity at which they experience depression and anxiety.[38] An interesting interplay exists between psychological and GI conditions; not only will GI conditions increase the likelihood of developing anxiety and depression but also they can be caused by psychological factors, such as stress and anxiety.[39]

In chronic medical conditions, IBH can play important roles, such as desensitizing before procedures to reduce anxiety, demystification, and explanation of outcomes. IBH, if introduced within a patient's care team quickly after diagnosis or even when no problem is present, can build rapport with the patient and family.[2] In most cases, this team will see the patient anytime they come to the clinic, be it for a specific concern with their diagnosis or a well-child visit. These multiple points of communication allow for better assessment of mental health and behavioral development of the patient.[2] Providers on this team can help assess changes in a patient's mood and behavior as well as provide consultation services and care coordination.[2]

MENTAL HEALTH DISORDERS
Tags: Attention-Deficit/Hyperactivity Disorder, Anxiety, Depression

Mental health disorders are lifetime conditions that have extensive impacts on individual's social well-being and physical health. Three common mental health disorders that have a high prevalence in childhood and adolescence include attention-deficit/hyperactivity disorder (ADHD), anxiety, and depression. Care for these patients is complicated and tends to require large amounts of follow-up visits for surveillance of symptom flares and maintenance of medical management. Because these patients are seen regularly, it is important to include IBH intervention in their health care plan, which may help in diagnosis of comorbid conditions, if not the initial diagnosis.

In 2014, it was estimated that 11% of all children have a diagnosis of ADHD,[40] with a steady increase in diagnoses over the past decade. ADHD symptoms can impact children's academic standings,[41] likely because of their impaired ability to concentrate on tasks during class times and also on social and interpersonal functioning outside the school environment (home and community). Individuals with ADHD have higher incidences of school absences because of expulsions and suspensions for their behaviors.[41,42]

It is estimated that by the age of 16 around 9.5% of patients exhibit symptoms of a depressive disorder in the United States[43] with an increased risk for suicidal thought processes and risky behaviors,[44] which can be detrimental to both physical and mental health.[45] At the same time, approximately 10% of all children by the age of 16 will experience an anxiety disorder,[43] and these individuals struggle with comorbid depression, conduct disorder, and substance use disorders.[43] In pediatric populations, these disorders are complicated by the fact that children are often unable to articulate their feelings and concerns accurately, which makes diagnosis difficult[43]; however, parents and caregivers are helpful informants on these issue for clinicians.[43]

Other disruptive disorders that could be a target for IBH intervention include the diagnoses of conduct disorder and oppositional defiant disorder. Estimates for these disorders are around 20% of individuals before they reach their 16th birthday,[43] and these disorders are often comorbid with the other mental health disorders described above.[43] When a child presents with any of the mental health conditions, it is important to rule out other underlying medical diagnoses that might be causing the symptoms.

An IBH consultant can be an integral member of a care team within a PCMH, identifying, diagnosing, and treating behavioral and mental health conditions. IBH specialists may due this through symptom and function assessment tools, assessing the patient's motivation to engage in treatment, helping families identify goals and possible solutions, providing guidance to community and institutional resources, and even engaging in short-term, brief psychosocial and behavioral interventions.

SUMMARY

Routine well-child visits in the primary care setting are implemented in order to ensure appropriate mental and physical development throughout a child's life. IBH can aid in this by identifying any early concerns or difficulties as well as provide resources and support when these issues first emerge, thus promoting the child's well-being.[2] There are many medical and mental health conditions that present in the primary care medical home that offer the opportunity for an IBH consultant to engage the patient and family. This can be especially helpful in the setting of psychosocial problems[27] and chronic conditions.[2] The consultant can serve many roles in screening, intervention, advocacy, and guidance, thus contributing to the child's overall well-being.

CLINICS CARE POINTS

- Routinely scheduled well-child visits are ideal to assess developmental progress, environmental health, behavior/psychosocial issues, and other parental concerns.[1] Delivering integrated behavioral health (IBH) in the primary care setting may aid in identifying any early concerns or difficulties in the above categories.[2]

- The patient-centered medical home[13] is an ideal location for coordinating mental health care. IBH can serve a variety of roles for the patient/family and the clinician, including anticipatory guidance, health promotion, mental health consultations, family support, and guidance to other resources.

- The incorporation of IBH helps caregivers normalize discussion of behavioral or emotional issues in a primary care setting and sets the stage for addressing mental health issues.[14]

- IBH consultants can also be involved in screening at each well-child visit for behavioral or mental health disorders using broad-based standardized tools, such as the Pediatric Symptom Checklist)[15] and Ages and Stages Questionnaire,[16] among others.

- Parental divorce or loss has a large impact on the social and behavioral development of a child during crucial stages of life. Children may experience problems that may include anxiety, depression, violence, anger, and regression of developmental milestones.[23] In this setting, IBH involvement can provide behavioral counseling, coping strategies, providing parental support and direction to appropriate ancillary resources.

- There is a significant positive impact of family support programs on changing parent behavior in order to prevent or improve early childhood behavioral problems.[26] IBH can aid in this process by providing the necessary resources or direct parental support.

- In chronic medical conditions, IBH can play important roles, such as desensitizing before procedures to reduce anxiety, demystification, and explanation of outcomes. IBH, if introduced within a patient's care team quickly after diagnosis or even when no problem is present, can build rapport with the patient and family.[2]

REFERENCES

1. Hagan JF, Shaw JS, Duncan P. Bright futures guidelines for health supervision of infants, children, and adolescents. 3rd edition. Elk Grove Village (IL): American Academay of Pediatrics. 2008.
2. Talmi A, Muther EF, Margolis K, et al. The scope of behavioral health integration in a pediatric primary care setting. J Pediatr Psychol 2016;41(10):1120–32.
3. van der Lee JH, Mokkink LB, Grootenhuis MA, et al. Definitions and measurement of chronic health conditions in childhood: a systematic review. JAMA 2007; 297(24):2741–51.
4. Meltzer H, Gatward R, Goodman R, et al. Mental health of children and adolescents in Great Britain. Int Rev Psychiatry 2003;15(1–2):185–7.
5. Hysing M, Elgen I, Gillberg C, et al. Chronic physical illness and mental health in children. Results from a large-scale population study. J Child Psychol Psychiatry 2007;48(8):785–92.
6. Lavigne JV, Faier-Routman J. Psychological adjustment to pediatric physical disorders: a meta-analytic review. J Pediatr Psychol 1992;17(2):133–57.
7. Asarnow JR, Rozenman M, Wiblin J, et al. Integrated medical-behavioral care compared with usual primary care for child and adolescent behavioral health: a meta-analysis. JAMA Pediatr 2015;169(10):929–37.

8. Combs-Orme T, Heflinger CA, Simpkins CG. Comorbidity of mental health problems and chronic health conditions in children. J Emot Behav Disord 2002;10(2): 116–25.

9. Pinquart M, Shen Y. Behavior problems in children and adolescents with chronic physical illness: a meta-analysis. J Pediatr Psychol 2011;36(9):1003–16.

10. Cohen P, Pine DS, Must A, et al. Prospective associations between somatic illness and mental illness from childhood to adulthood. Am J Epidemiol 1998; 147(3):232–9.

11. Orr DP, Weller SC, Satterwhite B, et al. Psychosocial implications of chronic illness in adolescence. J Pediatr 1984;104(1):152–7.

12. Olsson CA, Bond L, Johnson MW, et al. Adolescent chronic illness: a qualitative study of psychosocial adjustment. Ann Acad Med Singap 2003;32(1):43–50.

13. Jackson GL, Powers BJ, Chatterjee R, et al. Improving patient care. The patient centered medical home. A systematic review. Ann Intern Med 2013;158(3): 169–78.

14. Briggs-Gowan MJ, Horwitz SM, Schwab-Stone ME, et al. Mental health in pediatric settings: distribution of disorders and factors related to service use. J Am Acad Child Adolesc Psychiatry 2000;39(7):841–9.

15. Jellinek MS, Murphy JM, Robinson J, et al. Pediatric symptom checklist: screening school-age children for psychosocial dysfunction. J Pediatr 1988; 112(2):201–9.

16. Valleley R, Roane B. Review of ages & stages questionnaires: a parent-completed child monitoring system. In: Spies RA, Carlson JF, Geisinger KF, editors. The eighteenth mental measurements yearbook. 3rd edition. Lincoln (NE): Buros Center for Testing; 2010.

17. Sheldrick RC, Merchant S, Perrin EC. Identification of developmental-behavioral problems in primary care: a systematic review. Pediatrics 2011;128(2):356–63.

18. Sheldrick RC, Henson BS, Neger EN, et al. The baby pediatric symptom checklist: development and initial validation of a new social/emotional screening instrument for very young children. Acad Pediatr 2013;13(1):456–67.

19. Briggs RD, Stettler EM, Silver EJ, et al. Social-emotional screening for infants and toddlers in primary care. Pediatrics 2012;129(2):e377–84.

20. Atlas J. Test review of the children's depression inventory. In: Carlson Janet F, Geisinger Kurt F, Jonson Jessica L, editors. The nineteenth mental measurements yearbook. Lincoln (NE): Buros Institute of Mental Measurements; 2014.

21. Reynolds C, Richmond B. RCMAS-2: revised children's manifest anxiety scale title. Los Angeles (CA): Western Psychological Services. 2008.

22. Harold GT, Sellers R. Annual research review: interparental conflict and youth psychopathology: an evidence review and practice focused update. J Child Psychol Psychiatry 2018;59(4):374–402.

23. Cerel J, Fristad MA, Verducci J, et al. Childhood bereavement: psychopathology in the 2 years postparental death. J Am Acad Child Adolesc Psychiatry 2006; 45(6):681–90.

24. Amato PR, Keith B. Parental divorce and the well-being of children: a meta-analysis. Psychol Bull 1991;110(1):26–46.

25. Hickson GB, Altemeier WA, O'Connor S. Concerns of mothers seeking care in private pediatric offices: opportunities for expanding services. Pediatrics 1983; 72(5):619–24.

26. Kaminski JW, Valle LA, Filene JH, et al. A meta-analytic review of components associated with parent training program effectiveness. J Abnorm Child Psychol 2008;36(4):567–89.

27. Thomas R, Abell B, Webb HJ, et al. Parent-child interaction therapy: a meta-analysis. Pediatrics 2017;140(3). https://doi.org/10.1542/peds.2017-0352.
28. Kurtz BP, Abrams AN. Psychiatric aspects of pediatric cancer. Child Adolesc Psychiatr Clin N Am 2010;19(2):401–21.
29. Pettitt DJ, Talton J, Dabelea D, et al. Prevalence of diabetes in U.S. youth in 2009: the SEARCH for diabetes in youth study. Diabetes Care 2014;37(2):402–8.
30. Fagot-Campagna a, Pettitt DJ, Engelgau MM, et al. Type 2 diabetes among North American children and adolescents: an epidemiologic review and a public health perspective. J Pediatr 2000;136(5):664–72.
31. Delamater AM. Psychological care of children and adolescents with diabetes. Pediatr Diabetes 2009;10(Suppl 12):175–84.
32. Janssen I, Craig W, Boyce W, et al. Associations between overweight and obesity with bullying behaviors in school-aged children. Pediatrics 2004;113(5):1187–94.
33. Alegria Drury CA, Louis M. Exploring the association between body weight, stigma of obesity, and health care avoidance. J Am Acad Nurse Pract 2002; 14(12):554–61.
34. Strauss RS. Childhood obesity and self-esteem. Pediatrics 2000;105(1). https://doi.org/10.1542/peds.105.1.e15.
35. Akinbami LJ, Simon AE, Rossen LM. Changing trends in asthma prevalence among children. Pediatrics 2016;137(1):e20152354.
36. Moonie S, Sterling D, Figgs L, et al. The relationship between school absence, academic performance, and asthma status. J Sch Health 2008;78(3):140–8.
37. Alexander KL, Entwisle DR, Horsey CS. From first grade forward: early foundations of high school dropout. Sociol Educ 1997;70(2):87–107.
38. Chang L. Review article: epidemiology and quality of life in functional gastrointestinal disorders. Aliment Pharmacol Ther 2004;20(Suppl 7):31–9.
39. Levy RL, Olden KW, Naliboff BD, et al. Psychosocial aspects of the functional gastrointestinal disorders. Gastroenterology 2006;130(5):1447–58.
40. Visser SN, Danielson ML, Bitsko RH, et al. Trends in the parent-report of health care provider-diagnosed and medicated attention-deficit/hyperactivity disorder: United States, 2003-2011. J Am Acad Child Adolesc Psychiatry 2014;53(1): 34–46.e2.
41. Loe IM, Feldman HM. Academic and educational outcomes of children with ADHD. J Pediatr Psychol 2007;32(6):643–54.
42. LeFever GB, Villers MS, Morrow AL. Parental perceptions of adverse educational outcomes among children diagnosed and treated for ADHD: a call for improved school/provider collaboration. 2002;39(1).
43. Costello EJ, Mustillo S, Erkanli A, et al. Prevalence and development of psychiatric disorders in childhood and adolescence. Arch Gen Psychiatry 2003;60(8): 837–44.
44. Mojtabai R, Olfson M, Han B. National trends in the prevalence and treatment of depression in adolescents and young adults. Pediatrics 2016;138(6):e20161878.
45. Kessler RC, Berglund P, Demler O, et al. The epidemiology of major depressive disorder: results from the National Comorbidity Survey Replication (NCS-R). JAMA 2003;289(23):3095–105.

The Continuum of Intervention Models in Integrated Behavioral Health

Alexander W. Sullivan, BA[a], Sheryl Lozowski-Sullivan, MPH, PhD[b],*

KEYWORDS

- Integrated behavioral health models • Pediatric primary care
- Continuum of integration • Models of clinical collaboration • Integrated primary care

KEY POINTS

- Recommend communication between mental health and primary care providers via fax, telephone, electronic health record, and secure email at the least integrated level.
- Transdisciplinary mental and primary physical health in the same location with concurrent consultation, joint decision-making, and shared responsibility are accomplished with purposeful effort and funding at the most integrated level.
- Specialized training in the medical model for psychologists and social workers includes: population-based care; evidence-based brief interventions (eg, adherence to medical treatment, parenting, toileting); health and behavior codes, medical diagnostic codes; fast pace of primary care; and concise communications.
- Psychologists and social workers should seek integrated behavioral health positions in university, medical school, and progressive primary care settings.

Models of clinical collaboration between physical and mental health providers in the pediatric outpatient primary care setting fall along a continuum of integration of services and philosophies of care. Domains of integration include the physical office location, targeted patient population, level of professional adaptation to other professions' model of training, and the influence of current models of reimbursement (**Fig. 1**). Several authors have described a variety of models for clinical collaboration in pediatric primary care. Most of these authors do not favor the most prevalent model in the United States today, Independent Functions, based primarily on the disassociation of the patient's physical from their behavioral/mental health and sequelae that arise from this perspective of the mind-body/brain dualism. An analysis of those models is discussed with respect to where it falls on each continuum of integration.

[a] Department of Social Work, Wayne State University, 5447 Woodward Avenue, Detroit, MI 48202, USA; [b] Department of Pediatric and Adolescent Medicine, Western Michigan University, Homer Stryker MD School of Medicine, 1000 Oakland Drive, Kalamazoo, MI 49008-8071, USA
* Corresponding author.
E-mail address: sheryl.lozowski-sullivan@med.wmich.edu

Pediatr Clin N Am 68 (2021) 551–561
https://doi.org/10.1016/j.pcl.2021.03.001
0031-3955/21/© 2021 Elsevier Inc. All rights reserved.

pediatric.theclinics.com

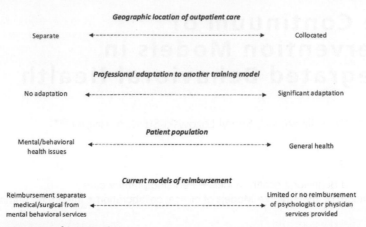

Fig. 1. Continuums of integration.

The two models currently most prevalent throughout the United States are geographically separate offices: Independent Functions and Indirect Consultation.

SEPARATE OFFICE LOCATIONS
Independent Functions

The most pervasive model in current medical practices is Independent functions[1] or Specialist-Generalist. In this traditional medical model, the psychologist/social worker (specialist[a]) provides consultation, diagnosis, and treatment of the referred patient at a separate office location. The pediatric physician (generalist) retains primary and over- all health responsibility for the patient. Communication between the physician and psychologist/social worker is typically in the form of written communications but may include telephone calls. The generalist approaches mental/behavioral health ser- vices similar to other specialist services, such as cardiac, orthopedic, surgical ser- vices. The patient returns to primary care after the presenting issue is stabilized and/or resolved. From a patient population perspective, this model targets those pa- tients for whom mental/behavioral health services are deemed to be needed by the physical health provider.

Fee-for-service reimbursement mechanisms favor this model because mental and behavioral health services are typically paid separately from medical/surgical ser- vices.[2] However, this reimbursement mechanism also limits the successful linkage to mental health services if the referred specialist provider is not paneled or partici- pating in the insurance network or if the specifics of the client's plan (ie, number of visits allowed, copayments/insurance, deductibles) insufficiently cover services or overly burden the client.

This model follows a traditional philosophy of mind-body/brain dualism; the artificial separation between physiology and psychology of the human.[3] Since the 1970s, an explosion of research reintegrates the "mind" and the brain illustrating the iterative processes between physical and mental health. The fields of behavioral medicine and later, clinical health psychology, emerged from these experimental findings.[3]

Research suggest the Independent Functions or Specialist-Generalist model do not sufficiently link clients to mental and behavioral health services. Approximately 15% of

---

[a] Clinical psychologists and medical social workers are the most common nonmedical mental health specialists in medical settings.

patients seek mental/behavioral health services on advice/referral from physicians. Low compliance may be systemic (ie, reimbursement system), geographic (distance from provider), or sociologic (ie, stigma of mental health).[4] The underlying assumption of the model is that these services are similar to other specialty services; however, the referral is not approached by patients like other specialty services, in that, 85% of patients do not follow physicians' advice for mental/behavioral health services.[4]

Another critical limitation is inherent in the divergent training of physicians, psychologists, and social workers. Physicians typically refer to other specialist pediatric physicians (neurology, cardiology, surgery, psychiatry) who have similar medical training. Differences in training and practice between the physician and psychologist/social workers may impede communication and understanding between physicians and mental health professionals.[3,4] There are several differences between the traditional work environments of psychologists/social workers and the pediatric primary care work environment.[5–8] These include different norms, practices, languages, and roles.[5–7] These issues may limit communication between the physician and psychologist through written and verbal contacts.

The Independent Functions or Specialist-Generalist model is currently the most pervasive model in the United States. However, there are barriers that limit linkage to services. Ultimately, when a patient engages with the referral, the style of communication between the providers may not serve the overall health needs of the patient well. Several theorists, dissatisfied with this model, offer alternatives to this model.

Indirect Consultation

Similar to the previously mentioned model, the Indirect Consultation[1] or Consultation places the pediatrician and psychologists/social worker typically in separate physical office spaces. In this model, the psychologist and social worker provide advice and/or information regarding behaviors, interpretation of test data, community resources, and so forth via telephone, case conferences, seminars, and other collaborative venues. Christophersen[9,10] provides a critical example through extensive research and training of primary care physicians in implementation of standardized treatment protocols (eg, behavioral compliance, compliance with medical procedures, sleep, eating and toileting). The physician maintains primary responsibility for the patient and seeks advice as needed from the psychologist/social worker. A primary advantage of this model is the robustness of service in the primary care setting with the existing service providers. Christophersen's version of this model is more integrated along the patient population continuum of care because pediatricians trained in several behavioral health treatment protocols can deliver a wide variety of common general health and behavioral solutions presented in the pediatrician office. Pediatricians serve as the de facto mental health professional and de facto psychiatrist because of the severe shortage of pediatric psychiatrists.[11]

The Indirect Consultation model is dependent on the ability of the physician to diagnose and treat the issue correctly. Physicians are in the position of seeking advanced training in treatment protocols, such as those in Christophersen's Pediatric Compliance,[10] which may stretch some pediatricians beyond their training and comfort in medicine to behavioral psychology. The physician's role expands, and they have discretion to request consultation with a psychologist/social worker. Unfortunately, the physician and the psychologist/social worker provide similar services and therefore may compete and/or refrain from consultation. Likewise, there are no mechanisms for psychologist reimbursement under the Independent Consultation model unless both are staff clinicians in a medical or university setting. For pediatricians in private practice, the time allocated for office visits limits their ability to provide such treatment protocols to families.

COLLOCATION MODELS

Five models integrate physicians and psychologists/social workers geographically in the same physical office space. These include: Collocated Specialty model, Consultation with Collocation,[12] Chronic Condition programs,[12] Collaborative Team,[1,12] and Reverse Collocation.[13] Increasing evidence suggests primary care providers are the most likely professionals to receive questions regarding behavioral or emotional concerns[1] and often do not have adequate time or skills to address such concerns.[2]

Collocated Specialty Model

This model involves the psychologist/social worker serving in the primary care clinic setting. The services are traditional mental/behavioral health and substance abuse services. The Collocated Specialty model requires little adaption for each provider because they perform independently, as specialist-generalist, simply in the same space. The proximity may facilitate a greater appreciation and understanding of the functions of the physician and/or psychologist, and it may increase opportunities for "curbside" or face-to-face case collaboration between physician and psychologist.[12] Psychologists on staff of medical schools are often training medical and psychology students concurrently using the Collocated Specialty model. Similarly, this model targets primarily those patients viewed by the pediatrician as needing specialty mental/behavioral health services. When children have mental/behavioral services needs that relate to a medical condition, the Health and Behavior procedure codes paired with International Classification of Diseases (ICD) diagnoses may be applicable and payable. These Common Procedural Terminology codes are paid from the medical benefits of the insurance subscriber rather than the mental health benefits but require that the patient does not have a Diagnostic and Statistical Manual Fifth Edition (DSM-5) diagnosis attributable to the services provided.[3]

Disadvantages of the Collocation Specialty are consistent with the two previous models in the inherent separation between physical health care and behavioral/mental health care also known as mind-body dualism.[3] The psychologist/social worker is not typically considered a core member of the primary care team but as an in-house specialist. The primary problem with this perspective is it fails to address the issue of misallocation of resources that exists in primary care today.[14] This often results in the same access problems that occur in noncollocated specialty behavioral/mental health care because the traditional 50-minute hour with each patient does not allow for more than seven to eight patients per day. This model is labor intensive for the on-site psychologist/social worker. Under this model, psychologists/social workers do not have the ability to serve large numbers of primary care patients and, as result, the psychologist/social worker tends to get referrals for the most difficult patients. The result is a heavy and difficult caseload for the in-house psychologist/social worker with only a small percentage of the population of patients accessing mental health care. Services remain focused on those in need of mental/behavioral health needs rather than general health, such as adherence with medical regimes, successful parenting, developmental changes, and so forth.[14–16]

Consultation with Collocation

Consultation with Collocation involves the psychologist/social worker located in the same office space as the physician, available for mental/behavioral health regardless of the type of issue. The design of the office space itself can restrict or foster integration of mental/behavioral health into primary care.[17] This can occur in the form of phone-in[18,19] or face-to-face consultation. Typically, the psychologist or social worker meets with 14 to 18 patients per day for brief problem-focused services, such as developmental questions, behavioral issues, school-related concerns.[12,15,18,19] The psychologist or social worker may schedule another brief visit or refer the patient to a community provider for more intensive treatment. This model is more fully integrated along the patient population continuum addressing more general health-related concerns and mental/behavioral issues rather than solely mental/behavioral issues.[18]

Access to behavioral/mental health services within the primary care setting[14,20] is an advantage of this model. It is estimated that three out of the five questions parents ask pediatricians involve behavioral concerns.[14,20] The most commonly addressed concern among parents was compliance/oppositional behaviors, which pediatricians view as the most challenging.[20] More than 50% of concerns pediatricians hear are behavioral.[14,20] Increased access to mental/behavioral health services may increase compliance with medical and psychological advice by services provided by a psychologist or social worker.[21] In addition, the stigma of seeking mental/behavioral care may be reduced by virtue of the mental health professional placement within the pediatric primary care setting.[14,22]

One disadvantage of this model is the nontraditional nature of the psychological services requiring increased training for the psychologist and social workers. This includes an understanding of the primary care setting as a "population-based care" wherein the goals include preventing illness through management of health risk factors, early detection, and so forth and managing illness through measuring, such as chronic medication management, palliative care, and so forth. Overall, primary care acts as the medical home and manages total patient care through referral to and coordination with various medical specialtles.[4] Psychologists/social workers must seek additional training in psychopharmacology, behavioral medicine, and health psychology.[6,7] They must also learn to accommodate to the fast pace of primary care in terms of time management and effective communications with patients and with physicians.[1,5,6] Psychologist/social workers need to develop a variety of time-efficient assessment and intervention skills in mental health, chemical dependency, behavioral medicine, and health psychology to address the varied needs of the primary care population.[6] Physicians are also required to understand the services provided by the psychologist/social worker and adapt their referral patterns from the traditional specialist-generalist training model.

Chronic Condition Programs

Like Consultation with Collocation, Chronic Condition programs are integrated on-site programs requiring that psychologists seek specialized training. Chronic Condition programs are also called "critical pathways," "clinical roadmaps," or "disease management" targeting patients with chronic conditions. Providers use standard treatment guidelines, care protocols, and processes for best clinical outcomes, such as management of pediatric diabetes.[9] Christophersen delineates techniques for improving compliance with medical regimes generally, including parent and patient education, written instructions, recoding symptoms accurately, and increased follow-up by medical professionals and parents.[8,9] In addition, chronic disease regimens include checklists, educational strategies, implementation of complex regimens, and monitoring of compliance and symptoms of disease. Chronic Condition programs require that the targeted condition is well represented in the specific primary care population and/or the implementation has a potential impact on service use or cost. Moreover, there should be one or more behavioral or pharmacologic treatments known to be effective for a given condition to target the condition.[21] The Reverse Colocation model[10] may fit within the Chronic Condition model because this model involves the primary care physician located within a mental health setting. Typically, this is a community mental health or predominately mental/behavioral health agency.

Strengths of the Chronic Condition program or model are the specialized services targeting specific conditions and the reimbursement for such services through Health and Behavior Common Procedural Terminology codes.[3,18] This model extends integration of the patient population from mental/behavioral health to more general chronic care patient needs. Limitations include advanced training, that is, psychologists/social workers must understand how to assess, monitor, and quantify clinical response for each visit.[3,4,7,8] Psychologists/social workers may also be in the position of administering and collecting all data related to such a program and adapt their traditional 50-minute session to much briefer visits.

Collaborative Team

The most integrated model along the continuums of integration described previously is the Collaborative Team model or True Collaboration or Primary Care Behavioral Health Model.[4,21] This model is characterized by joint decision-making and shared responsibility among physicians, psychologists, and in many cases other professionals.[2,4] Examples of these models are available in pediatric inpatient care (eg, pediatric oncology team, intensive feeding team) and in medical school training programs but few collaborative team models exist in the pediatric outpatient community setting. In one such model, established by Chapel Hill Pediatric Psychology in 1973, a private psychological practice collocated with a community medical pediatric practice.[22,23] It emphasizes prevention and early intervention rather than treatment of psychopathology, and exemplifies programmatic collaboration by providing call-in hours twice a week for 2 hours, a walk-in service, parent education groups and materials, developmental screening, assessment and intervention (as educator, advocate, treatment provider, and case manager), and community collaboration (eg, sex education). Variations of this model have been implemented in federally funded community health centers (Cherokee Health Systems and Hawaii Integrated Healthcare Project II), primary care clinics within the US Air Force[24] and Army, and some Veterans Administration clinics.[25-27] Several large private health care organizations, such as the Group Health Cooperative of Puget Sound and Kaiser Permanente, use the Primary Care Behavioral Health Model. A broad variety of services are requested in primary mental health care including consultation and follow-up, triage, community resource referral, treatment compliance, relapse prevention, case management, patient-physician consultation, provider consultation, team building, and on-demand consultation.[12,21-23] Within this model the psychologist or social worker is called the "Behavioral Health Consultant." The Behavioral Health Consultant sees the patient for 15 to 30 minutes for one to four visits after the primary care provider when a problem is identified. Assessments in this setting focus on functioning (rather than diagnostics), symptom elimination, and functional restoration.[28-30] Such services have been found to be valued by the primary care physician in the assessment, treatment, and monitoring of primary care patients.[28,29] The most effective empirically supported pediatric treatments are conducive to the primary care setting because of their preventive potential. Examples of such evidence-based interventions include: behavioral parent training for attention-deficit/hyperactivity disorder; behavior modification for enuresis and encopresis[14]; cognitive behavior therapy for distress because of medical procedures; effective use of time out; and dealing with tantrums, obesity, stomach and headaches, and school issues.

An advantage of this model is the potential for medical cost offset; receipt of more appropriate services that avoid or reduce more costly services[20,28] and improved pediatric treatment outcomes.[28,31] Studies evaluating medical cost offset coincide with the evolution of the health care delivery system from fee-for-service to managed care.[31] Medical cost offset is realized in the current health delivery system when short-term focused behavioral health interventions are incorporated into the primary care delivery system. This is accomplished through an improved fit between care patients seek in primary care and services delivered that may, in fact, improve overall patient satisfaction with medical and behavioral/mental health services. Moreover, 90% of patients in the primary care setting who present with physical and behavioral/mental health issues follow medical advice when such services are onsite, whereas 15% of patients seek noncollocated specialty mental/behavioral health service referrals.[31] More recently, several studies support cost-effective and evidence-based interventions for depressive symptoms, pain management, and cognitive behavioral therapy for insomnia.[31]

Another advantage of this model is the integration of behavioral health as a part of the process of general health care and primary health promotion.[2,19,20] Behavioral/ mental health care is more likely perceived by patients as a routine aspect of health care[6,20,21] and may return to the primary care psychologist for periodic care rather than initiating psychotherapy and terminating when the issue is resolved.[6] In addition, several studies indicate integrated mental health care into primary care leads to better outcomes and cost savings.[28,31,32] Examples of improved outcomes for pediatric patients include child behavior problems, attention-deficit/hyperactivity disorder and adolescent depression,[20] and reduced emergency department visits.[33,34] An additional benefit of this model to providers is shared expertise of a variety of different disciplines (ie, medicine, nursing, psychology, social work) in clinical management, and the opportunity for providers to expand their professional skills and perspectives. For example, a psychologist may attend psychopharmacology training to gain an appreciation for the neurologic foundations of pharmacologic therapy.[28]

Members of the care team must learn to share responsibility, communicate, be flexible in terms of their role, and negotiate professional territory. Time requirements and personnel costs for such a model may also be a limitation. The psychologist's role in pediatric primary care is to support the primary medical service as consultant, assessor or treating provider.[5] Services provided are short-term, intense, and problem-focused aimed at the presenting problem, and a premium is placed on prompt follow-up after a referral. Psychologist/social workers and physicians also need to maintain mutual respect for each other's expertise and boundary issues that differ in their respective training models, which require effective communication and adaptation to nontraditional roles and practices. Psychologists in primary care settings work in an environment that is largely "physician driven and physician controlled" within the constraints of business, government regulation, and economics.[34] Physicians wield greater influence in numbers of professionals and relative power, which places psychologists and social workers in positions of comparatively limited influence. Psychologists are often in the position of garnishing respect through their clinical acumen and contributions and their ability to be collegial.

A major limitation noted by Drotar[1] is the critical leadership component. Without strong leadership that fosters shared decision-making, care teams can decompose into indecision and dissension. Likewise, leadership may act autocratically and fragment a team.[1] Drotar's comments in 1995 underscores the importance of professional flexibility and willingness to integrate other perspectives into clinical primary care.

Six models of clinical and care collaboration fall along a continuum of most to least integrated. These models reflect contemporary research and implementation between mental health providers and physicians in pediatric primary care. The models emphasize the interactions and relationships of physicians and psychologists (and other professionals); however, a different perspective is provided by Drotar.[1] This is a Systems Model[1] or Psychologist as Community Collaborator,[2] which examines the broader context in which collaborative relations occur. His focus on the needs and interventions of the broad community, nonetheless, do not fit in current reimbursement mechanisms.[2] Typically, Systems Model programs are developed by mental health and community partners, preventive in nature (eg, sex education, nicotine education), and integrated into the existing educational or health care systems.[2,35] Each model offers advantages and limitations in terms of professional adaptation and training, patient access to behavioral/mental health services, reimbursement mechanisms, and the focus of services.

The wisdom of integrating behavioral health in pediatric primary medical care settings is described in the literature over several decades.[1–8,17,19,21,30,31] Conceptual underpinnings of these models date back to the emergence of different mental health providers (ie, child welfare, psychology, social work, developmental pediatrics, psychiatry). Several models of integrated behavioral health are successful but require changes in professionals' perspectives, training, delivery of care, physical location, arrangement within the physical space, and communication. The components of integrated models that maximize cost-effectiveness and access have yet to be fully delineated[36–39] and achieved; value-based reimbursement[5,18,40–42] for integrated behavioral health in pediatric primary care is imperative to the success of these models.

CLINICS CARE POINTS

- Models of clinical collaboration in the integrated behavioral health pediatric primary care setting range from least integrated (verbal or written communications) to most integrated (Collaborative Team).
- Each model has advantages and limitations in terms of professional adaptation and training, patient access to behavioral/mental health services, reimbursement dilemmas and service focus on psychopathology or population-based preventive care.
- Conceptual underpinnings of these models date back to the emergence of the various mental health provider types; child welfare, psychology, social work, developmental pediatrics, psychiatry.
- Several models of integrated behavioral health are successful such as, pediatric specialist psychologist/social workers in University-based children's hospitals whereas, integrated behavioral health in pediatric primary care is limited and models vary widely.
- Value-based reimbursement for integrated behavioral health in pediatric primary, utilizing decades of research on mind-body connections is requisite to population-based mental health services in primary care.

DISCLOSURE

The authors have no affiliations to disclose.

REFERENCES

1. Drotar D. Consulting with pediatricians: psychological perspectives. New York: Plenum Press; 1995.

2. Black M, Nabors L. Behavioral and developmental problems of children in primary care: opportunities for psychologists. In: Frank R, McDaniel S, Bray J, editors. Primary care psychology. Washington, DC: American Psychological Association; 2004. p. 189–207.
3. Belar CD, Deardorff WW. Clinical health psychology in medical settings: A practitioner's guidebook. Washington, DC: American Psychological Association; 1995.
4. Strosahl K. The integration of primary care and behavioral health: type II changes in the era of managed care. In: Cummings N, O'Donohue W, Hayes S, et al, editors. Integrated behavioral healthcare: positioning mental health practice with medical/surgical practice. New York: Academic Press; 2001. p. 45–70.
5. Strosahl K, Robinson P. Behavioral health consultation and primary care: lessons learned. J Clin Psychol Med Settings 2009;16:58–71.
6. Clay DL, Stern M. Pediatric psychology in primary care. In: James L, Folen R, editors. The primary care consultant: the next frontier for psychologists in hospitals and clinics. Washington, DC: American Psychological Association; 2005. p. 155–72.
7. Burg MA, Oyama O. The behavioral health specialist in primary care: skills for integrated practice. New York: Springer; 2016.
8. Dobmeyer AC, Rowan AB, Etherage JR, et al. Training psychology interns in primary behavioral health care. Prof Psychol Res Pract 2003;34(6):586–94.
9. Christophersen E, Mortweet SL. Treatments that work with children: empirically supported strategies for managing childhood problems. Washington, DC: American Psychological Association; 2001.
10. Christophersen E. Pediatric compliance: a guide for the primary care physician (Critical issues in developmental and behavioral pediatrics). New York: Plenum; 1994.
11. Findling RL, Stepanova E. The workforce shortage of child and adolescent psychiatrists: is it time for a different approach? J Am Acad Child Adolesc Psychiatry 2018;57(5):300–1.
12. O'Donohue WT, Byrd MR, Cummings NA, et al. The case for integrated care: coordinating behavioral health care with primary care. In: O'Donohue WT, Byrd MR, Cummings NA, editors. Behavioral integrative care: treatments that work in the primary care setting. New York: Routledge; 2005. p. 1–14.
13. Shackelford JR, Sirna M, Mangurian C, et al. Descriptive analysis of a novel health care approach: reverse colocation—primary care in a community mental health "home. Prim Care Companion CNS Disord 2013;15(5):1–11.
14. Blum NJ, Friman PC. Behavioral pediatrics: the confluence of applied behavior analysis and pediatric medicine. In: Austin J, Carr J, editors. Handbook of applied behavioral analysis. Oakland, CA: Context Press; 2000. p. 161–86.
15. Hunter CL, Goodie JL, Oordt MS, et al. Integrated behavioral health in primary care: step-by-step guidance for assessment and intervention. 2nd edition. Washington, DC: American Psychological Association; 2017.
16. Gatchel R, Oordt M. Clinical health psychology and primary care: practical advice and clinical guidance for successful collaboration. Washington, DC: American Psychological Association; 2003.
17. Gunn R, Davis M, Hall J, et al. Designing clinical space for the delivery of integrated behavioral health and primary care. J Am Board Fam Med 2015; 28(Suppl 1):S52–62.
18. Cummings NA, O'Donohue WT, Cummings JL. The financial dimension of integrated behavioral/primary care. J Clin Psychol Med Settings 2009;16:31–9.

19. Collins C, Hewson D, Munger R, et al. Evolving models of behavioural health integration in primary care. New York: Milbank Memorial Fund; 2010.
20. Kolko D, Campo D, Kilbourne A, et al. Collaborative care outcomes for pediatric behavioral health problems: a cluster randomized trial. Pediatrics 2014;133: 381–92.
21. Strohsal K, Robinson P. The primary care behavioral health model: applications to prevention, acute care and chronic condition management. In: Kessler R, Stafford D, editors. Collaborative medicine case studies: evidence in practice. New York: Springer; 2008. p. 85–95.
22. Schroeder CS, Gordon BN. Assessment and treatment of childhood problems: a clinician's guide. 2nd edition. New York: The Guilford Press; 2004.
23. Schroeder CS, Smith-Boydston JM. Assessment and treatment of childhood problems: a clinician's guide. 3rd edition. New York: The Guilford Press; 2017.
24. Wilson PG. The Air Force experience: integrating behavioral health providers into primary care. In: Frank RG, McDaniel SH, Bray JH, et al, editors. Primary care psychology. Washington, DC: American Psychological Association; 2004. p. 169–85.
25. Felker BL, Chaney E, Rubenstein LV, et al. Developing effective collaboration between primary care and mental health providers. Prim Care companion J Clin Psychiatry 2006;8:12–6.
26. Post EP, Metzger M, Dumas P, et al. Integrating mental health into primary care within the Veterans Health Administration. Families, Syst Health 2010;28:83–90.
27. Post EP, Van Stone WW. Veterans Health Administration primary care-mental health integration initiative. North Carolina Med J 2008;69:49–52.
28. Njoroge W, Hostutler CA, Schwartz BS, et al. Integrated behavioral health in pediatric primary care. Curr Psychiatry Rep 2016;18:1–8.
29. Ramanuj P, Ferenchik E, Docherty M, et al. Evolving models of integrated behavioral health and primary care. Curr Psychiatry Rep 2019;21:1–12.
30. Robinson P, Reiter J. Behavioral consultation and primary care: a guide to integrating services. New York:: Springer; 2007.
31. Robinson P, Reiter J. Behavioral consultation and primary care: a guide to integrating services. New York: Springer; 2014.
32. Asarnow JR, Rozenman M, Wiblin J, et al. Integrated medical-behavioral care compared with usual primary care for child and adolescent behavioral health: a meta-analysis. JAMA Pediatr 2015;169:929–37.
33. Estee S, Wickizer T, He L, et al. Evaluation of the Washington State Screening, brief intervention, and referral to treatment project: cost outcomes for Medicaid patients screened in hospital emergency departments. Med Care 2010;48:18–24.
34. Serrano N, Prince R, Fondow M, et al. Does the primary care behavioral health model reduce emergency department visits? Health Serv Res 2018;53(6): 4529–42.
35. Garcia-Shelton L, Leventhal G. Psychology's adaptation to medical schools, teaching hospitals and academic medical centers: the role of academic medicine organizations. J Clin Psychol Med Settings 2005;12:221–34.
36. Jacobsen PB, Prasad R, Villani J, et al. The role of economic analyses in promoting adoption of behavioral and psychosocial interventions in clinical settings. Health Psychol 2019;38:680–8.
37. Knapp P, Foy JM. Integrating mental health care into pediatric primary care. J Am Acad Child Adolesc Psychiatry 2012;51:982–4.

38. Heath B, Wise RP, Reynolds KA. A review and proposed standard framework for levels of integrated healthcare. Washington, DC: SAMHSAHRSA Center for Integrated Health Solutions; 2013.
39. Yonek J, Lee C, Harrison A, et al. Key components of effective pediatric integrated mental health care models: a systematic review. JAMA Pediatr 2020; 174:487–98.
40. O'Donnell AN, Williams M, Kilbourne AM. Overcoming roadblocks: current and emerging reimbursement strategies for integrated mental health services in primary care. J Gen Intern Med 2013;28(12):1667–72.
41. Strosahl K. Identifying and capitalizing on the economic benefits of integrated primary behavioral health care. In: Cummings N, O'Donohue W, Ferguson K, editors. The impact of medical cost offset on practice and research: making it work for you. Reno, NV: Context Press; 2002. p. 57–90.
42. Miller BF, Miller BF, Mendenhall TJ, et al. Integrated primary care: an inclusive three-world view through process metrics and empirical discrimination. J Clin Psychol Med Settings 2009;16:21–30.

The Behavioral Health Consultant

Roles and Responsibilities

Heidi Joshi, PsyD[a],*, Pilar Corcoran-Lozano, MA[b]

KEYWORDS

- Primary care behavioral health (PCBH) model • Pediatrics • Integrated primary care
- Behavioral health consultation

KEY POINTS

- Behavioral health integration within pediatric primary care considers the behavioral health consultant as a primary provider on the team that allows for destigmatization while increasing accessibility and availability to scarce mental health services.
- The behavioral health consultant engages in brief consultations referred to as "warm hand-offs" in the primary care setting, to screen, detect, prevent, and provide appropriate interventions related to mental health and general well-being.
- For integrative services to continue and expand, the lack of uniformity of reimbursement pushes for additional empirical evidence to further support their established benefit, such as the cost-effectiveness of prevention and providing brief intervention. In addition, there is a need for psychology and social work programs to incorporate training and education of operating within a primary care environment with the specific needs of a pediatric clinic.

INTRODUCTION

Because of the growing scarcities in behavioral health resources such as psychiatric and psychological interventions, solutions including integrating behavioral health services into primary care become more important.[1,2] Evidence is mounting for the fact that integrating behavioral health services into primary care settings destigmatizes mental health care, can serve a broader range of patients, promotes better access, and capitalizes on the concept of prevention implicit in primary care.[3,4] For the purposes of this article, primary care is defined in part as the initial contact and a comprehensive continuity care for individuals with any health concern not limited by the origin of the problem, such as biological, behavioral, or social, the organ system, or diagnosis.[5] In addition, primary care includes health promotion and maintenance, disease

[a] John Muir Health Family Medicine Residency, 1450 Treat Boulevard Suite 320, Walnut Creek, CA 94597, USA; [b] John F. Kennedy University, John F. Kennedy School of Psychology at National University, 100 Ellinwood Way, Pleasant Hill, CA 94523, USA
* Corresponding author.
E-mail address: Heidi.Joshi@johnmuirhealth.com

Pediatr Clin N Am 68 (2021) 563–571
https://doi.org/10.1016/j.pcl.2021.02.002
pediatric.theclinics.com

prevention, education and counseling for the patient, and diagnosis and treatment of acute and chronic illnesses.[5]

A continuum exists regarding the level of behavioral health integration in primary care.[6,7] At one end of the continuum, primary care providers refer to a behavioral health therapist in the community. However, the interaction between the providers is absent and no integration of records or treatment plan occur,[8] which is often known as specialty mental health. In the middle of this continuum is the concept of a colocated model. This model entails a more traditional mental health construct with the service colocated in the same treatment space as the medical office. In this colocated model, medical records and treatment plans may or may not be integrated, but patients often have to schedule an appointment on a different day than their medical visit and adhere to the workings of the specific behavioral health provider's schedule. On the other end of the continuum is a fully integrated model where the behavioral health consultant (BHC) is considered a primary provider on the care team[9] and interventions are brief and solution focused.[10] All documentation completed by either the medical provider or the behavioral health provider are located within the same chart and an integrated treatment plan is also used.[8] A model that exemplifies this full integration well is the Primary Care Behavioral Health (PCBH) model.[1,4,9–11]

PRIMARY CARE BEHAVIORAL HEALTH MODEL

The PCBH model is a team-based, fully integrated model that aims to increase accessibility and availability of behavioral health services in primary care by focusing on a population of patients.[12,13] BHC is a generalist; they can work across the lifespan with diverse medical and mental health presentations. Overall, PCBH aspires to promote and further improve the primary care team's comfort and capability to treat and manage behavioral health- and biopsychosocial-related health conditions within primary care.[13,14]

Population Health

Population health can be accomplished by using unique patient appointment types such as group visits.[9] These visits are where providers see several patients at a time with the same medical condition. Providers see several adolescents with depression, for example, and benefit from consolidating these visits, by saving time and increasing productivity. Most importantly, however, these group visits offer avenues to increase support and education for these adolescents. Another strategy the providers in the PCBH model use to maximize the population focus is to integrate themselves into all aspects of clinic flow. Many PCBH providers will engage in activities such as giving "health talks" in waiting rooms while patients are waiting to be called for their appointments. These Health Talks can be on topics such as stress management, parenting issues, or how to make lifestyle changes. They are talks that can benefit most of the people in the waiting rooms. BHCs often have handouts and posters in patient rooms regarding specific and pertinent issues such as sleep disturbances, and some will even offer an appointment with the BHC for every patient in the practice regardless of their presenting problems. This normalizes the service and further destigmatizes behavioral health care.[9] The primary goal of these strategies is for the BHC to focus on the entire patient population in the medical practice, thereby increasing access to services and decreasing stigma.

Screening

Practices using the PCBH model avail themselves of screening tools for issues such as depression, substance use, or anxiety; this increases the likelihood that patients with these concerns will be detected and appropriate interventions can be sought.[15–17] The idea is screening of all patients, not singling out any particular group, at various intervals of care such as once per year. Particular patients needing specific attention and intervention are brought to the attention of the BHC and others on the care team. The BHC can then assist the care team in providing further assessment and appropriate intervention. The benefit is the patient experiencing this screening and intervention process have not had to find another provider outside the primary care setting, nor have they been singled out for their specific concern through the referral process. There has been no waiting for an appointment outside the clinic for several weeks or worry that a provider will not be found who can help them with their concerns. This screening and intervention process is conducted by the same clinic and the same care team that presumably is familiar with the patient.

Warm Hand-Off

Another crucial work of the PCBH model is the use of "warm hand-offs."[18] The BHC can be introduced to the patient by this one important avenue. The medical provider, who presumably has a longer-term relationship with the patient introduces the BHC to the patient during their visit with the medical provider. This brief introduction offers advantages such as transference or organizational transference; the feeling the patient holds toward the medical provider/organization is transferred onto the BHC, potentially allowing rapport to be easier and/or quicker to develop. The assumption of this concept is that patients would think "if my doctor thinks this person can help me, then I'll see them" and "I trust my doctor, I trust this new person." The availability of the BHC to engage in these warm hand-offs and often see patients during that same visit as their medical providers goes a long way to increasing access to behavioral health services for patients and increases provider and patient satisfaction.[19,20] Incidentally, as noted in a qualitative review by Hunter and colleagues, provider and patient satisfaction was the largest advantage noted in studies done of the PCBH model.[20] Consequently, barriers of health care coverage restrictions, limited behavioral health resources/providers, long-wait times for services, transportation issues, and patient's follow through with referrals[14] strengthen the need for application of the PCBH model and warm hand-offs. Using warm hand-offs promotes the availability of same-day appointments with BHCs, accessibility of behavioral health services, and also assists in intervening quickly in behavioral health matters. In fact, the authors would argue that they would not see the same success in satisfaction and patient engagement without warm hand-offs, which are vital to the success of the PCBH model.

Another notable advantage is the rapid response clinicians and patients receive through the warm hand-off process.[21] This rapid response can help both medical providers and patients feel attended to and lessen barriers to behavioral health treatment.[21] Having BHCs on the care team can foster providers' understanding of behavioral health issues and how to manage them.[22] All in all, the population focus, access to rapid care, and the ability to have a behavioral health expert on the care team are all benefits for both patients and providers.

Limitations of the Primary Care Behavioral Health Model

The PCBH model, by design, relies on licensed mental health professionals.[9] This model has advantages such as being able to bill for their services but also has its limitations. BHCs, such as psychologists and social workers, are not specifically trained to work in primary care environments after graduating from their respective training programs.[1,23] As such, more specific training is needed to assist these practitioners to work in the fast-paced world of primary care and help them focus on the brief assessment and intervention skills so important in the PCBH model.[23] Therefore, continued workforce development is vital to the success of the PCBH model.[1]

Another difficulty practices using the PCBH model encounter is that of reimbursement. The lack of uniformity regarding payment structures makes it difficult to use this model in many areas of the country. The fee-for-service world, which is especially prevalent in the United States, presents many barriers for getting appropriately paid especially in the realm of integrated behavioral health services, and. this specifically puts practices who use the PCBH model at a marked disadvantage.[12,19,24] Consequently, alternative payment models are needed to fully realize the possible financial benefits to behavioral health integration.[12,24] Behavioral health services are typically "carved out," and often the expectation of insurance companies is that these treatments will be done in specialty mental health settings that are, by their nature, not appropriate for primary care settings. In addition, billing for mental health visits is typically done by time and by diagnosis. Primary care behavioral health visits, by necessity, are shorter in length, and the interventions are often connected with medical diagnosis as well as mental health ones. Ideally, payment models would reflect the brief, integrated nature of the PCBH model necessary in primary care and behavioral health integration. Insurance companies would pay for behavioral health integration in primary care in order to reduce costs associated with mental health issues. What can be difficult for practices to illustrate to insurance companies is that much of the cost savings is on the back end with prevention and early detection of mental health issues. Moreover, lower rates of hospitalizations and better adherence to medication regiments also save money in the long run.[4,20]

Another limitation of the model is that of superficiality. For the small percentage of patients seen in primary care with extremely severe mental health issues, the PCBH model may not be enough to manage their disorders. Disorders such as extreme personality or psychotic disorders, to name a couple, would be difficult to manage in a primary care setting—this is not to say that these patients do not get served in primary care. It is, rather, more helpful to have a specialty mental health provider and psychiatrist assist in their mental health care. The PCBH model does not take a deep dive into interventions. Because of the utilization of a consultative approach meant to focus on increasing access and brief interventions, specialty mental health can often be a more appropriate choice for caring for severely mentally ill patients.

PRIMARY CARE BEHAVIORAL HEALTH AND PEDIATRICS

Approximately 21% of young people have a mental health diagnosis but only 1/5 of them get treatment.[15] In addition, 50% of all lifetime mental health disorders begin by the age of 14 years.[25] It is also known that intervening as early as possible in a child's life can help children continue on their normal trajectory of development or assist a child in returning to a more normal one.[26] Individuals living with mental illness have a life expectancy of 15 to 20 years less than those without mental illness.[27] Integrating behavioral health in pediatric practices has been shown to assist in early detection and prevention of developmental and behavioral health concerns.[15,26,28] Studies have already shown the positive behavioral changes and lowered levels of parental stress for children with disruptive behavioral concerns who had access to an integrated behavioral health provider.[28] Similarly, Oppenheim and colleagues, in their article regarding the Substance Abuse and Mental Health Services administration's (SAMHSA's) project where grantees used 5 evidence-based strategies, aimed to improve the social, emotional, and community outcomes for at-risk children and their families.[26] One such strategy was integration of behavioral health in pediatric practices and another was screening for neurodevelopmental and behavioral health concerns.[26] The preliminary data from this project show that, as a result of implementing these strategies in their grant projects, there were improvements in individual child outcomes, such as an increase in behavioral and social skills. Better family outcomes including lower rates of parental stress and depression were also noted. In addition, provider outcomes of more knowledge regarding social and emotional development along with community outcomes such as better collaboration between service providers were found.[26] These preliminary data support utilization of the PCBH model in pediatrics clinics, as behavioral health integration is implicit in the PCBH model along with screening for developmental and behavioral health concerns.[9]

Research confirms that pediatric primary care providers do conduct behavioral health interventions. However, there is limited time allotted per visit, providers view their role in behavioral health as limited, and providers have a range of comfort, capability, and experience in behavioral health screening, diagnosing, treating, and interventions.[14] Medical schools and medical trainings provide a limited range of brief instruction related to behavioral and mental health.[29] However, there are efforts and calls for action for schools and training sites to increase education related to the latter.[29,30] Moreover, primary care providers indicated a need for consultation and "reassurance that they are adequately addressing pediatric behavioral health needs."[14] BHC can close this gap in learning by providing training and education and conducting joint visits with pediatric providers to further foster their ability to screen, treat, and intervene behavioral health concerns presenting in their examination rooms.[14]

A key aspect of pediatric practices, especially here in the United States, is that of the well-child visit. Well-child visits are about preventing issues and being proactive with children's health care. The goals of well-child visits include health promotion, disease prevention through routine vaccinations and education, early detection and treatment of disease, and parental guidance for the optimization of the child's emotional and intellectual development.[31] Given the importance of prevention in well-child visits, the PCBH model is seen as a natural expansion of this prevention focus. Because of the heightened access to behavioral health providers in the model, screening can happen along with brief interventions as needed. Just like in well-child visits, PCBH visits often entail screening for specific symptoms such as substance abuse (Substance Abuse and Mental Health Services Administration's Screening, Brief Intervention and Referral to Treatment [SBIRT]), depression (Patient Health Questionnaire [PQA]), anxiety, behavioral and psychosocial concerns (Pediatric Symptom Checklist [PSC]).[15,32] In the PCBH model, if a child screens positive during the well-child visit, the BHC can assist the child, family, and medical provider in obtaining a more specific diagnosis and appropriate treatment, often in the same examination space as the medical visit. The utilization of expedient and convenient clinically appropriate screening measures and intervention techniques goes a long way toward prevention and early detection of mental health problems in children, adolescents, and their families. Utilization of a BHC during a well-child visit allows for a biopsychosocial and whole-person approach to care.

The PCBH model destigmatizes behavioral health care by integrating BHCs into the medical context.[8,28] In doing so, it acknowledges the interconnection of both physical and mental health and allows for many to connect with a behavioral health provider for the first time. Ideally it introduces the patient to a warm, friendly, and welcoming experience of behavioral health, concluding that behavioral health is important as our physical health. Furthermore, this model allows for confidentiality, as patients can be seen by both medical and behavioral health providers within the same location and same visit. Patients in the waiting room may be presenting for a well-child visit, vaccines, or behavioral interventions for attention-deficit/hyperactivity disorder and no one would know.[8] The authors would argue that destigmatizing behavioral health care is even more important for children and teens, as they are not often the decision-makers regarding their treatment. If the parents or guardians feel comfortable with the process of behavioral health treatment, children and teens are much more likely to be given the opportunity for care. Also, in pediatric health care, access to behavioral health treatment is also significantly lacking.[8] This void is much wider in rural health settings.[8] The PCBH model directly addresses this resource deficit through its ability to see patients in their primary care provider's practices and on the same day as their medical providers. There is no wait time to see a specialty mental health provider and no referral needed to get an assessment or brief intervention.

FUTURE DIRECTIONS

There is a significant deficit in both the depth and breadth of the research of the PCBH model. Limited randomized trials exist regarding the PCBH model.[20] Partly, this is because of the difficulties in researching model fidelity.[21] The literature, for example, describes a range as to the length of a PCBH patient visit. The range, according to Mauksch, is between 15 and 40 minutes.[21] This leaves the question: what is the appropriate length of a PCBH visit? Does the length of the visit have any effect on the outcome for patients or providers? Also, adherent in the PCBH model is measurement of health outcomes or functional status. According to the literature, BHCs rarely do any formal measure of patient functional status but tend to document this more informally.[21] Many BHCs and developers of the PCBH model believe the model tends to focus on "behavioral medicine" issues such as health behavior changes and chronic diseases. In actuality, most providers of the PCBH model tend to see patients dealing foremost with depression and anxiety.[33] This makes sense when considering the accessibility of mental health resources for the primary care physician and patient through the integration of a BHC. An additional fidelity issue to consider is that warm hand-offs often look different depending on the provider and clinic setting.[21] More research is warranted on the outcomes of patient engagement and model fidelity based on a formulized and structured approach to warm hand-offs.

The suggestions of focusing future research on specific elements of the PCBH model in order to determine issues such as length of visits, structure of warm hand-offs, and other important variables would help to improve model fidelity and thereby improve PCBH research overall.[21]

Perhaps the most important limitation facing the PCBH model is that of a lack of an appropriate and consistent payment structure. Therefore, payment reform is needed on many health care fronts. Behavioral health care is no exception. Continuing to think about ways to help practices and providers who use integrated behavioral health is essential if the PCBH model and others like it can continue. More thought and research, however, regarding other value-added additions BHCs make in primary care is also crucial. Looking at issues such as the BHC role in cost reduction from lowering readmittance rates to the hospital, examining further the connections between teens who participate in services by a BHC and lowered rates of depression, and improved levels of functioning continue to be warranted. By continuing to expand the research done regarding the PCBH model in pediatric and adult settings and working toward innovative payment reform, the PCBH model and other models of primary care behavioral health integration can realize their full potential.

SUMMARY

The PCBH model is in a unique position to increase much needed access to primary care behavioral health services through innovative constructs such as warm hand-offs and the utilization of a consultative approach.[9] This population-based model with its solution-focused interventions provides an avenue to assist patients with immediate and affective assessment and intervention resources right in their primary care clinics. This unique approach is especially important in reaching children, adolescents, and their families due to the ongoing mental health shortage in this population. This model also is primed to meet the important detection and prevention needs of pediatric populations using screenings. As such, it behooves pediatric practices to take a closer look at the feasibility and acceptability of the PCBH model for their settings.

CLINICS CARE POINTS

- Behavioral Health Consultants are encouraged to be integrated in well-child visits to screen, prevent and conduct appropriate treatment related to emotional and mental health.
- Commonly seen in primary care, screening by Behavioral Health Consultants may encompass substance use (Screening, Brief Intervention and Referral to Treatment [SBIRT]) depression (Patient Health Questionnaire [PHQ-A]), anxiety, behavioral and psychosocial concerns (Pediatric Symptom Checklist [PSC]).
- Indicated as a need by primary care providers, the Behavioral Health Consultant can provide education, training, and in-vivo learning to strengthen a providers (whole-person) practice.

DISCLOSURE

The authors have nothing to disclose.

REFERENCES

1. Serrano N, Cordes C, Cubic B, et al. The state and future of the primary care behavioral health model of service delivery workforce. J Clin Psychol Med settings 2017. https://doi.org/10.1007/s10880-017-9491-1.
2. Grazier KL, Smiley ML, Bondalapati KS. Overcoming barriers to integrating behavioral health and primary care services. J Prim Care Community Health 2016;7(4):242–8.
3. Miller-Matero LR, Dubaybo F, Ziadni MS, et al. Embedding a psychologist into primary care increases access to behavioral health services. J Prim Care Community Health 2015;6(2):100–4.
4. Robinson PJ, Strosahl KD. Behavioral health consultation and primary care: lessons learned. J Clin Psychol Med Settings 2009;16(1):58–71.
5. AAFP. Primary Care [web page]. 2017. Available at: www.aafp.org/about/policies/all/primary-care.html. Accessed April 1, 2020.
6. Chapman E, Chung H, Pincus HA. Using a continuum-based framework for behavioral health integration into primary care in New York State. Psychiatr Serv 2017;68(8):756–8.

7. Wedding D, Mengel M. Models of integrated care in primary care settings. In: Haas LJ, editor. Handbook of primary care psychology. New York: Oxford University Press; 2004. p. 47–60. Chapter xxi, 639 pages.

8. Njoroge WFM, Hostutler CA, Schwartz BS, et al. Integrated behavioral health in pediatric primary care. Curr Psychiatry Rep 2016;18(12):106.

9. Robinson PJ, Reiter JT. Behavioral consultation and primary care: a guide to integrating services. New York (NY): Springer Science + Business Media; 2007. p. 481. Chapter xxv.

10. Dobmeyer AC. Conducting the behavioral health consultation appointment. Clinical health psychology series BT- psychological treatment of medical patients in integrated primary care. Washington, DC: American Psychological Association; 2018. p. 41–51. Chapter xi, 197 Pages.

11. Ogbeide SA. Review of Integrated behavioral health in primary care: Step-by-step guidance for assessment and intervention (Second edition). Fam Syst Health 2017;35(3):391.

12. Ader J, Stille CJ, Keller D, et al. The medical home and integrated behavioral health: advancing the policy agenda. Pediatrics 2015;135(5):909–17.

13. Reiter JT, Dobmeye AC, Hunter CL. The primary care behaviorall health (PCBH) model: an overview and operational defination. J Clin Psychol Med Settings 2018; 25:109–26.

14. Conners EH, Arora P, Blizzard AM, et al. When behavioral health concerns present in pediatric primary care: Factors influencing provider decision-making. J Behav Health Serv Res 2018;45(3):340–55.

15. Blucker RT, Jackson D, Gillaspy JA, et al. Pediatric behavioral health screening in primary care: a preliminary analysis of the pediatric symptom checklist-17 with functional impairment items. Clin Pediatr 2014;53(5):449–55.

16. Jacobson J. Behavioral health screening in children. Am J Nurs 2015;115(7): 19–20.

17. Mulvaney-Day N, Marshall T, Downey Piscopo K, et al. Screening for behavioral health conditions in primary care settings: a systematic review of the literature. J Gen Intern Med 2017. https://doi.org/10.1007/s11606-017-4181-0.

18. Berge JM, Trump L, Trudeau S, et al. Integrated care clinic: Creating enhanced clinical pathways for integrated behavioral health care in a family medicine residency clinic serving a low-income, minority population. Fam Syst Health 2017; 35(3):283–94.

19. Gouge N, Polaha J, Rogers R, et al. Integrating behavioral health into pediatric primary care: implications for provider time and cost. South Med J 2016; 109(12):774–8.

20. Hunter CL, Funderburk JS, Polaha J, et al. Primary care behavioral health (PCBH) model research: current state of the science and a call to action. J Clin Psychol Med settings 2017. https://doi.org/10.1007/s10880-017-9512-0.

21. Mauksch L, Peek CJ, Fogarty CT. Seeking a wider lens for scientific rigor in emerging fields: The case of the primary care behavioral health model. Fam Syst Health 2017;35(3):251–6.

22. Ratzliff A, Phillips KE, Sugarman JR, et al. Practical approaches for achieving integrated behavioral health care in primary care settings. Am J Med Qual 2017; 32(2):117–21.

23. Dobmeyer AC, Hunter CL, Corso ML, et al. Primary care behavioral health provider training: systematic development and implementation in a large medical system. J Clin Psychol Med Settings 2016;23(3):207–24.

24. Zivin K, Miller BF, Finke B, et al. Behavioral health and the comprehensive primary care (CPC) initiative: findings from the 2014 CPC behavioral health survey. BMC Health Serv Res 2017;17(1):612.

25. NAMI. Mental Health by the numbers. Available at: https://www.nami.org/learn-more/mental-health-by-the-numbers. Accessed April 1, 2020.

26. Oppenheim J, Stewart W, Zoubak E, et al. Launching forward: the integration of behavioral health in primary care as a key strategy for promoting young child wellness. Am J Orthop 2016;86(2):124–31.

27. Thornicroft G. Physical health disparitites and metnal illness: the scandal of premature mortality. Br J Psychiatry 2011;199:441–2.

28. Kolko DJ, Perrin E. The integration of behavioral health interventions in children's health care: services, science, and suggestions. J Clin child Adolesc Psychol 2014;43(2):216–28.

29. Smith RC. Educating trainees about common mental health problems in primary care: a (not so) modest proposal. Acad Med 2011;86:e16.

30. Smith RC, Laird-Fick H, D'Mello D, et al. Addressing mental health issues in primary care: an initial curriculum for medical residents. Patient Educ Couns 2014; 94:33–42.

31. Consolini DM. Health Supervision of the Well Child: Merck Sharp & Dohme Corp., a subsidiary of Merck & Co., Inc; 2017. Available at: http://www.merckmanuals.com/professional/pediatrics/health-supervision-of-the-well-child/health-supervision-of-the-well-child. Accessed April 1, 2020.

32. Hacker KA, Penfold R, Arsenault L, et al. Screening for behavioral health issues in children enrolled in Massachusetts Medicaid. Pediatrics 2014;133(1):46 54.

33. Beehler GP, Lilienthal KR, Possemato K, et al. Narrative review of provider behavior in primary care behavioral health: how process data can inform quality improvement. Fam Syst Health 2017;35(3):257–70.

Funding and Billing for Integrated Behavioral Health Care

Keshav Patel, MS[a,b,*], Roger W. Apple, PhD[a,b,c], Jessica Campbell, BS[a,b,d]

KEYWORDS

• Integrated behavioral health care • Funding • Billing • Coding • Cost-effective

KEY POINTS

• Integrated behavioral health care (IBHC) improves patient satisfaction and outcomes.
• IBHC programs have numerous financial barriers, including billing and coding requirements along with low reimbursement rates.
• When properly implemented, behavioral health consultants allow medical providers to see more patients and therefore indirectly increase the clinic revenue.
• We need more definitive models of successful IBHC to effectively incorporate it into clinics.

INTRODUCTION

The Institute of Healthcare Improvement has identified 3 goals that they wish to pursue, known as the Triple Aim. The Triple Aim consists of improving patient outcomes, decreasing cost, and increasing the quality of patient satisfaction.[1-3] Integrated behavioral health care (IBHC) improves patient outcomes, decreases cost, and increases patient satisfaction.[4-6] For example, children and adolescents treated with IBHC were 66% more likely to have better outcomes than children and adolescents treated with the usual care.[5] It has become increasingly evident that IBHC must be incorporated in the US health care system. However, the financial aspects of IBHC are greatly debated and not fully understood.[6-8] In this article, the authors discuss the funding and billing components of IBHC.

No disclosures necessary for any of the authors.
[a] Western Michigan University Homer Stryker MD School of Medicine, 300 Portage Street, Kalamazoo, MI 49007, USA; [b] Pediatric Psychology Subspecialty, Department of Pediatric and Adolescent Medicine, 1000 Oakland Drive, Kalamazoo, MI 49008; [c] Department of Pediatric and Adolescent Medicine, WMed Pediatric Autism Center, 1000 Oakland Drive, Kalamazoo, MI 49008; [d] Western Michigan University, 1903 W Michigan Avenue, Kalamazoo, MI 49008, USA
* Corresponding author. Western Michigan University Homer Stryker MD School of Medicine, Kalamazoo, MI.
E-mail address: keshav.patel@med.wmich.edu

DEFINITION

Several different definitions of IBHC exist. In this article, the authors define IBHC as integrated and coordinated care between the medical professional and behavioral health consultant (BHC). The BHC may be a social worker, psychologist, or another qualified professional. The type of provider is not crucial, but psychologists are the most qualified for IBHC.[9,10] Psychologists generally receive the most comprehensive training to support brief therapies and interventions necessary for IBHC.

An extensive literature search was done using the following databases: PsychInfo, PubMed, and Medline. Literature was sought out for integrated behavioral health, outpatient pediatrics, and behavioral health consultants. While reviewing the literature, it became clear that many investigators define IBHC in many different ways. Also, IBHC is a relatively recent health service and continues to work to define itself and its function in health care.

PEDIATRIC POPULATION

According to multiple studies, 20% of children have a behavioral health disorder at some point in their lives, but 70% to 80% of these children do not receive any services for the behavioral health disorder.[10,11] The first 5 years are especially important for the mental health and wellness of a child.[12] Many mental health problems arise at a young age and can progressively worsen with age. By treating pediatric patients with IBHC, we can prevent these complications from worsening and reduce the associated health care costs. For example, a pediatric patient with mental health concerns that are not addressed may develop major depressive disorder, which ultimately will increase the cost of health care and lead to a much lower quality of life for this individual.

WESTERN MICHIGAN UNIVERSITY SCHOOL OF MEDICINE

Western Michigan University School of Medicine is running IBHC in their outpatient pediatric clinic. Within this clinic, BHCs begin their day by reviewing the pediatric outpatient schedule in the electronic medical record to identify patients who may benefit from IBHC. The BHC schedules a separate appointment with these patients, who already have an appointment with a medical provider, so that the BHC note is easily identifiable and to ensure that IBHC services can be billed. If the BHC bills under the medical provider, the note does not show up as easily on the patient's chart review or list of appointments. The prescheduled appointments are seen by the BHC as initial assessments and are the first time a patient has seen the BHC. However, not all patients who may benefit from IBHC can be identified by reviewing the chart. During visits, physicians also identify patients who may benefit from IBHC and use a warm hand-off to allow the patient to see the BHC. BHCs also attend well-child visits to introduce IBHC to the parents. During these visits, the BHC is usually asked to discuss developmental milestones.

The outpatient pediatric clinic uses doctoral clinical and counseling psychology students to make their services more cost-effective. In Michigan, psychology student interns can bill for Medicaid services under the supervision of a fully licensed psychologist. When a patient has a non-Medicaid insurance plan, the supervising fully licensed psychologist will see the patient.

FUNDING

Substance Abuse and Mental Health Services Administration (SAMHSA) has provided many opportunities for IBHC through the Primary and Behavioral Health Care

Integration program. As of March 2017, SAMHSA planned to give $2 million in grant funding to 11 IBHC programs for up to 5 years.[13] Several other grants are available to support IBHC. Grants are a great way to initiate IBHC until it can be sustained on its own. The financial sustainability of IBHC once the funding ends is a key problem discussed in this article.

Most hospitals or practices engaged in IBHC have received grant funding to start the integration. However, after the grant funding ends, hospitals have a tough time sustaining the costs related to IBHC.[7,9] Most health care payments are based on Fee for Service (FFS). FFS encourages hospitals to do more procedures rather than focusing on patient outcomes. Rather than FFS, payments should be based on patient outcomes. Because the direct billing of the BHC is minimal, it is hard for hospitals to justify IBHC.[6,7] However, if the shift occurs from FFS to outcomes-based payment, IBHC would be encouraged because it leads to better patient outcomes in the long run.[4-6]

Cardiovascular disease and many other chronic diseases have a huge mental health component.[14] Half of the geriatric population with chronic diseases has depression.[15] Depression can significantly affect the outcomes of patients with other chronic diseases.[16] For example, if IBHC was implemented, diabetic individuals could be treated more efficiently for depression, and this could end up reducing the long-term costs related to diabetic complications, such as surgery and amputations. Similarly, IBHC could help lower costs associated with many other chronic diseases. A key point here is that the hospital itself does not save money, but rather the payer will save money by avoiding these long-term costs. Because IBHC is such a huge benefit to the payers, Medicare, Medicaid, and private insurers should switch its reimbursement rates to better incorporate IBHC. If insurance companies reimburse BHCs with higher rates, they will encourage IBHC and improve long-term outcomes for patients, which will end up saving money for these insurance companies in the long run.

PHYSICIAN RELATIONSHIP

If IBHC cannot be justified from the BHC billing directly,[6,7] we can also argue that BHCs enable the physician to bill more, allowing for greater profits long term.[17,18] BHCs can decrease the time the physician has to see the patient in several ways. BHCs can complete the medication agreements for patients taking controlled substances. BHCs can gather history on patients with psychiatric problems before the physician encounter and then convey the pertinent information to the physician. BHCs can return phone calls to patients with psychiatric concerns, meet with patients to discuss end-of-life issues, and perform anticipatory guidance along with many other tasks. For well-child visits, BHCs can administer the M-Chat and Vanderbilt, along with other assessments. We hope that BHCs can be financially self-sustainable. However, if the billing is not enough to justify their salary, BHCs can perform a wide variety of actions in the health care setting to improve the efficiency of the physician and indirectly justify their salary.

In one study, pediatricians only billed 1 specific code for behavioral-only visits, whereas more than 10 different medical-only codes were billed.[18] Behavioral-only visits required approximately 20 minutes of their time, whereas medical visits required 8 minutes. The compensation was significantly lower for the behavioral concerns. In this scenario, IBHC could have many positive effects. Many pediatricians may not delve into the behavioral health concerns that the BHC will address. Also, IBHC allows the pediatrician to save time and focus on the medical aspects, whereas the BHC can focus on mental health concerns. The pediatrician may be able to see that 20-minute behavioral-only visit in 8 minutes, and the BHC can address the behavioral health concerns. In this manner, the pediatricians will be able to see more patients in the same amount of time, increasing their revenue.[18]

In one primary care clinic model, there were approximately 0.7 BHCs for every 3 physicians.[7] For effective IBHC, the number of BHCs needed for each physician is quite low and the cost to hire a BHC is low compared to other providers. By allowing the physician to see more patients, BHCs improve the cost-effectiveness of health care.

One particular study analyzed a pediatric primary care clinic in a rural area. The researchers analyzed the days that the integrated BHC was present and compared them with the days that the BHC was not present.[17] This clinic used 5 primary care providers, 4 physicians, and 2 nurse practitioners. On days that the BHCs were present, doctors saw 42% more patients, and the practice generated $1142 more in revenue compared with days that the BHCs were not present. Also, providers spent 2 minutes less across all patients on days that the BHCs were present. The money was not generated directly through the BHCs, but rather indirectly from the additional revenue the medical providers were able to generate. One limitation of this study is that the BHCs were doctoral students, rather than accomplished BHCs with prior experience. The authors believe that with experienced BHCs, the practice would generate more revenue due to more efficient care. Nonetheless, this study shows the potential benefits of IBHC that primary care clinics all around the United States could benefit from.[17]

When a patient does not show up, the practice loses a considerable amount of time and money. In IBHC, the medical provider is colocated with the BHC, which proves beneficial when comparing the no-show rates of different practices. With IBHC, primary care clinics will have lower no-show rates, which will lead to increased revenue.[19] Also, the BHC is often able to meet with the patient after the medical provider is finished; this saves the patient time because they no longer have to make an extra trip to see the BHC. In addition, studies have shown that the wait time for patients was decreased in IBHC.[17]

BARRIERS

The BHC salary is usually not justified based on their individual reimbursements.[7] Insurances and other payers could resolve this manner, by restructuring their payment methods. More codes should allow the BHC to directly bill the insurance, along with higher compensation. Another challenge with IBHC is the lengthy documentation required for both billing and coding. Instead of wasting their valuable time with documentation, it would be more efficient if the BHCs and physicians could spend more time seeing patients.[6]

It is difficult for primary care practices to develop an optimal financial model due to several factors. One key barrier is the variation in state laws. Because different states may have different laws, the IBHC model has to be optimized according to each state.

Another challenge may be disagreements between the BHC and the medical provider. This challenge is inevitable in medicine; however, protocols can be put into place to establish a team-based approach that takes into account all of the different opinions and strives to come up with the best integrated decision possible. Another challenge is that the integrated BHC is entering a clinic with medical providers, which is a cultural change, and the BHC might feel isolated.[20] BHCs may feel more welcome if multiple BHCs are present. Although this may be feasible at larger institutions, many small clinics will only need one BHC.

Another significant barrier is appointment scheduling. BHCs may have a hard time managing the scheduled and spontaneous appointments. The BHC may have a scheduled appointment at 1:00 PM; however, the medical provider may encounter a patient at 1:00 PM who requires IBHC. It is important to establish a coordinated system that allows the BHC a balance between scheduled appointments and emergent concerns.[20] Unfortunately, there is a shortage of BHCs. In one study, the wait time for BHCs was 2 to 3 months.[10] Many geographic regions may lack access to BHCs, so it may be crucial to increase the number of BHCs in order to combat the increasing demand.

BILLING AND CODING

BHCs include psychologists, social workers, and various other mental health workers. Traditionally, BHCs would bill under Health and Behavioral Assessment (HBA) codes, which are a subset of the current procedural terminology (CPT) codes. However, HBA codes can only be used to bill patients who have a physical health diagnosis.[21] HBA codes cannot be used when a patient has a psychiatric diagnosis, but they can be used if the behavioral, emotional, or social problems affect a physical health problem. The HBA codes are used because they do not require obtaining a history, examination, or making a medical decision, which are all part of the evaluation and management services. Evaluation and management services increase the workload and thus have a higher fee. BHCs may not use an HBA code if the evaluation and management service is provided to the patient on the same day, if they are conducting psychological testing, or if the patient is completing forms or questionnaires without face time with the BHC.[21] The BHC may have to request the medical provider to change the primary referral reason or add another secondary diagnosis in order to comply with billing and coding, which adds unnecessary difficulty to their jobs. Often, BHCs may treat patients without billing for their services due to coding restrictions.

Psychologists are allowed to use CPT codes when treating patients with a physical health problem.[21] The patient can still have a mental health diagnosis; however, the CPT code would be used if the psychologist is addressing a physical health problem (**Table 1**). Although Medicare reimburses for the CPT codes, private insurers may not. BHCs can prevent health problems; however, CPT codes cannot be used until the patient is diagnosed with a physical health problem. The 2020 HBA and Health Behavioral Intervention (HBI) codes not only increased the number of codes that BHCs can bill but also significantly increased reimbursement rates. As of this time, it is unclear if the new codes will make BHCs financially sustainable on their own. Although this is a step in the right direction, the authors believe more codes and higher reimbursement rates are needed for optimization of IBHC.

At many academic institutions, there is a relative value unit (RVU) requirement. RVUs are used to determine the value of a medical service. The total number of RVUs may be used as a measure of productivity for the medical provider or BHC.[23] At academic institutions, psychologists or other BHC providers may have RVU requirements. RVU is not equivalent to billing. Certain codes may bill a lot but have a relatively low RVU or vice versa. In the pediatric outpatient setting at Western Michigan University, the BHCs are held to RVU requirements. However, at a nearby health center, the providers depend on billing and are not restricted based on the RVUs. The HBA code 96150 requires a medical diagnosis and has RVUs attached to it. However, the Mental Health Assessment code H0031, which is based on a mental health diagnosis, has no RVUs attached to it. Both codes provide a similar compensation; however, one code does not have any RVUs attached to it. If the BHC providers have RVU requirements, this may create an additional burden even if the BHCs are directly billing enough to sustain the IBHC.

	Table 1 Health behavioral assessment and intervention services codes[22]	
CPT	Description	Work Relative Value Units
Health Behavioral Assessment Services		
96156	Health behavioral assessment or reassessment	2.10
Health Behavioral Intervention Services		
96158	Health behavioral intervention, face to face (30 min)	1.45
+ 96159	Each additional 15 min	0.50
Group Intervention (2 or more patients)		
96164	Health behavioral intervention, face to face (30 min)	0.21
+96165	Each additional 15 min	0.10
Family Intervention with Patient Present		
96167	Health behavioral intervention, family present, face to face (30 min)	1.55
+96168	Each additional 15 min	0.55
Family Intervention without Patient Present		
96170	Health behavioral intervention, family present, face to face (30 min)	1.50
+96171	Each additional 15 min	0.54

Derived from the American Psychological Association 2020 Health Behavior Assessment and Intervention Services Web Page.

In the past, reimbursement rates did not even cover the cost of the BHC. Several clinics in an Oregon study only had a 30% return on the services that were billable.[6] These low reimbursement rates make it difficult for hospitals to justify IBHC, because it is not directly profitable in the current health care system. Individual states and insurance companies have their own guidelines and rules, adding another layer of complexity. The current system is confusing, extremely complicated, and has many restrictions for BHCs. If we want IBHC to be incorporated in hospitals and clinics all over the United States, we need to adjust the billing and coding requirements for BHCs. The 2020 HBA and HBI codes are a step in the right direction, but as of now, it is unclear if the new codes and higher reimbursement rates are enough to implement IBHC in clinics all over the United States.

SUMMARY

At this current point, almost all health care professions recognize the need for integrated health care. IBHC allows the care of an individual as a whole, rather than treating each of the patient's symptoms and problems separately. IBHC significantly improves long-term patient outcomes. Although everyone agrees that IBHC is beneficial, there is a great debate on the financial sustainability of IBHC. Many IBHC programs may be started with grant funding; however, the funding is limited, and once the funding ends, the IBHC may no longer be financially sustainable. The billing and coding requirements often prevent BHCs from financial self-sustainability. The low reimbursement rates make it difficult to justify IBHC, because it is not directly profitable in the current health care system. The 2020 HBA and HBI codes are a step in the right direction, but as of now, it is unclear if the new codes and higher reimbursement rates are enough to directly justify the BHC's salary. When properly implemented, BHCs allowed medical providers to see more patients and spend less time on each patient. Therefore, BHCs can be indirectly justified through additional revenue through medical providers. In addition, if payers focus on long-term outcomes rather than FFS, IBHC will gain more support.

More definitive models of successful IBHC are needed. With these models, the authors hope to analyze both the mistakes and strengths of each IBHC attempt in order to come up with guidelines that can serve as a framework for primary care practices wishing to incorporate BHCs. There are numerous theories as to how the hospital or primary care clinics should structure IBHC. However, because IBHC is relatively new, more examples are needed before finding the best method of integration.

SUMMARY

- IBHC improves patient outcomes and satisfaction. Children and adolescents treated with IBHC were 66% more likely to have better outcomes than children and adolescents treated with the usual care.[5]
- IBHC programs may be started with grant funding; however, programs may not be financially sustainable once the funding ends.
- The billing and coding requirements, along with low reimbursement rates often prevent BHCs from financial self-sustainability in IBHC.
- The 2020 HBA and HBI codes are a step in the right direction, but as of now, it is unclear if the new codes and higher reimbursement rates are enough to directly justify the BHC's salary.
- IBHC may be financially sustainable if payment switches from FFS to outcomes-based payments.
- When properly implemented, BHCs allowed medical providers to see more patients and spend less time on each patient.
- IBHC is relatively new and we need more definitive models of successful IBHC to effectively incorporate IBHC into clinics.

CLINICS CARE POINTS

- Twenty percent of children have a behavioral health disorder at some point in their childhood, but most of these children do not receive any services for the behavioral health disorder.[10,11]
- When treated with IBHC, children and adolescents were 66% more likely to have better outcomes than children and adolescents treated with usual care.[5]
- IBHC lowers no-show rates in primary care clinics, which leads to increased revenue.[19]
- If there is a shift from FFS to outcomes-based payment, IBHC would be encouraged because it leads to better patient outcomes in the long run.[4-6]
- For effective IBHC, the number of BHCs needed per physician is low, and the cost to hire a BHC is low compared to other providers.[7]

REFERENCES

1. Institue for Health Care Improvement. Institute for Healthcare Improvement: The IHI Triple Aim [Internet]. IHI Triple Aim Webpage. 2016. Available at: http://www.ihi.org/Engage/Initiatives/TripleAim/Pages/default.aspx. Accessed January 14, 2018.

2. Berwick DM, Nolan TW, Whittington J. The triple aim: care, health, and cost. Health Aff 2008;27(3):759–69. Available at: http://content.healthaffairs.org/cgi/doi/10.1377/hlthaff.27.3.759. Accessed March 9, 2018.

3. Seow H-Y, Sibley LM. Developing a dashboard to help measure and achieve the triple aim: a population-based cohort study. BMC Health Serv Res 2014;14(1): 363. Available at: http://bmchealthservres.biomedcentral.com/articles/10.1186/1472-6963-14-363. Accessed March 9, 2018.

4. Laderman M. Behavioral health integration: a key component of the triple aim. Popul Health Manag 2015;18(5):320–2. Available at: http://online.liebertpub.com/doi/10.1089/pop.2015.0028. Accessed January 14, 2018.

5. Asarnow JR, Rozenman M, Wiblin J, et al. Integrated medical-behavioral care compared with usual primary care for child and adolescent behavioral health. JAMA Pediatr 2015;169(10):929. Available at: http://www.ncbi.nlm.nih.gov/pubmed/26259143. Accessed January 14, 2018.

6. Kroening-roché J, Hall JD, Cameron DC, et al. Integrating behavioral health under an ACO global budget : barriers and progress in Oregon. Am J Manag Care 2017;23(9):e303–9.

7. Monson SP, Sheldon JC, Ivey LC, et al. Working toward financial sustainability of integrated behavioral health services in a public health care system. Fam Syst Health 2012;30(2):181–6. Available at: http://www.ncbi.nlm.nih.gov/pubmed/22563727.

8. Muse AR, Lamson AL, Didericksen KW, et al. A systematic review of evaluation research in integrated behavioral health care: operational and financial characteristics. Available at: https://search-proquest-com.ezproxy.med.wmich.edu/docview/1910839233/fulltextPDF/E8F56E85DA72404EPQ/1?accountid=160899. Accessed January 19, 2018.

9. Chaffee B. Financial models for integrated behavioral health. [Internet]. The primary care toolkit: practical resources for the integrated behavioral care provider. p. 19–30. 2009. Available at: http://ovidsp.ovid.com/ovidweb.cgi?T=JS&PAGE=reference&D=psyc6&NEWS=N&AN=2008-16078-003. Accessed January 19, 2018.

10. Adams CD, Hinojosa S, Armstrong K, et al. An innovative model of integrated behavioral health: school psychologists in pediatric primary care settings. Adv Sch Ment Health Promot 2016;9(3–4):188–200. Available at: https://www.tandfonline.com/doi/full/10.1080/1754730X.2016.1215927. Accessed March 9, 2018.

11. Dabrow S, Adams C, Takagishi J, et al. An Innovative Model of Integrated Behavioral Health (IBH): School Psychologists in Continuity Clinic. Acad Pediatr 2016; 16(6):e48. Available at: http://linkinghub.elsevier.com/retrieve/pii/S1876285916302698. Accessed June 5, 2018.

12. Oppenheim J, Stewart W, Zoubak E, et al. Launching Forward : The Integration of Behavioral Health in Primary Care as a Key Strategy for Promoting Young Child Wellness. Available at: https://www.researchgate.net/profile/Whitney_Stewart3/publication/297746822_Launching_forward_The_integration_of_behavioral_health_in_primary_care_as_a_key_strategy_for_promoting_young_child_wellness/links/57729d7608ae2b93e1a7c8a8/Launching-forward-The-integration-of-behavioral-health-in-primary-care-as-a-key-strategy-for-promoting-young-child-wellness.pdf. Accessed March 9, 2018.

13. SAMHSA is accepting applications for up to $110 million in grants promoting integration of primary and behavioral health care | SAMHSA - Substance Abuse and

Mental Health Services Administration. Available at: https://www.samhsa.gov/newsroom/press-announcements/201703231100. Accessed May 11, 2018.

14. Mental Health and Heart Health. Available at: http://www.heart.org/HEARTORG/HealthyLiving/StressManagement/HowDoesStressAffectYou/Mental-Health-and-Heart-Health_UCM_438853_Article.jsp#.WlwkSUtG2_s. Accessed January 14, 2018.

15. Guan S, Fang X, Hu X. Factors influencing the anxiety and depression of patients with dilated cardiomyopathy. Int J Clin Exp Med 2014;7(12):5691–5. Available at: http://www.ncbi.nlm.nih.gov/pubmed/25664092. Accessed January 14, 2018.

16. Zhang Y, Chen Y, Ma L. Depression and cardiovascular disease in elderly: Current understanding. J Clin Neurosci 2018;47:1–5. Available at: http://www.ncbi.nlm.nih.gov/pubmed/29066229. Accessed January 14, 2018.

17. Gouge N, Polaha J, Rogers R, et al. Integrating behavioral health into pediatric primary care: implications for provider time and cost. South Med J 2016;109(12):774–8. Available at: http://sma.org/southern-medical-journal/article/integrating-behavioral-health-pediatric-primary-care-implications-provider-time-cost. Accessed February 17, 2018.

18. Meadows T, Valleley R, Haack MK, et al. Physician "Costs" in Providing Behavioral Health in Primary Care. Clin Pediatr (Phila) 2011;50(5):447–55. Available at: http://journals.sagepub.com/doi/10.1177/0009922810390676. Accessed December 15, 2017.

19. Guck TP, Guck AJ, Brack AB, et al. No-show rates in partially integrated models of behavioral health care in a primary care setting. Fam Syst Health 2007;25(2):137–46. http://doi.apa.org/getdoi.cfm?doi=10.1037/1091-7527.25.2.137. Accessed February 18, 2018.

20. Davis M, Balasubramanian BA, Waller E, et al. Integrating behavioral and physical health care in the real world: early lessons from advancing care together. J Am Board Fam Med 2013;26(5):588–602. Available at: http://www.ncbi.nlm.nih.gov/pubmed/24004711. Accessed February 18, 2018.

21. Billing, Reimbursement And Financing | IBHP. Available at: http://www.ibhpartners.org/get-started/procedures/billing-reimbursement-and-financing/. Accessed January 14, 2018.

22. Services A. 2020 Health Behavior Assessment and Intervention Services CPT® Codes & Descriptions CPT® Code # Descriptor Health Behavior Assessment Services. 2019. Available at: https://nam03.safelinks.protection.outlook.com/?url=https%3A%2F%2Fwww.apaservices.org%2Fpractice%2Freimbursement%2Fhealth-codes%2Fdescriptors-with-rvus.pdf&data=04%7C01%7Cr.mayakrishnan%40elsevier.com%7C4e1238592d22408b313708d8e3e86f5c%7C9274ee3f94254109a27f9fb15c10675d%7C0%7C0%7C637509936254166490%7CUnknown7CTWFpbGGZsb3d8ey JWIjoiMC4wLjAwMDAiLCJQIjoiV2luMzIiLCJBTiI6Ik1haWwiLCJXVCI6Mn0%3D%7C1000&sdata=IyVEYz96A0ynZjJInFdZR2ykpEkxM%2Fd7IEQ6Hg5PoIA%3D&reserved=0. Accessed December 18, 2019.

23. Storfa AH, Wilson ML. Physician productivity. Am J Clin Pathol 2015;143(1):6–9. Available at: https://academic.oup.com/ajcp/article/143/1/6/1760679. Accessed June 5, 2018.

Behavioral Health in Primary Care

Brief Screening and Intervention Strategies for Pediatric Clinicians

Rachel A. Petts, PhD[a],*, Scott T. Gaynor, PhD[b]

KEYWORDS

- Integrated behavioral health • Pediatrics • Brief interventions • ADHD • Anxiety
- Depression • Disruptive behavior • Substance use

KEY POINTS

- Pediatric primary care clinicians are tasked with managing and treating most childhood behavioral health problems, including disruptive behavior disorders, attention-deficit/hyperactivity disorder, anxiety, depression, and substance use.
- Screening for these behavioral health problems should occur in primary care and can help facilitate early intervention and referral.
- Regardless of access to an on-site behavioral health provider, pediatric clinicians can provide brief, evidence-based psychosocial interventions for behavioral health problems in addition to typical primary care management practices.
- Clear referral guidelines help identify children who may need specialty treatment outside of the primary care setting.

BACKGROUND

Primary care is the key setting in which individuals obtain mental health treatment, making it the de facto mental health system in the United States.[1–3] For youth, this means that pediatricians, family medicine physicians, and other pediatric primary care providers (eg, nurse practitioners and physician assistants) are required to manage the majority of pediatric psychological concerns, including mental health disorders, subthreshold behavioral/emotional symptoms, and behavioral factors that contribute to health (all described hereafter as behavioral health problems or concerns[4,5]). Moreover, due to a lack of pediatric psychiatrists, these pediatric providers

The authors have no conflicts of interest to disclose.
[a] Department of Psychology, Wichita State University, 1845 Fairmount Street, Wichita, KS 67260, USA; [b] Department of Psychology, Western Michigan University, 1903 West Michigan Avenue, Kalamazoo, MI 49008, USA
* Corresponding author.
E-mail address: rachel.petts@wichita.edu

Pediatr Clin N Am 68 (2021) 583–606
https://doi.org/10.1016/j.pcl.2021.02.010

also must prescribe and manage most psychotropic medications.[6,7] With numerous patients to see a day and only a relatively brief amount of time to spend with each, it is a challenge for providers to find the time to address all the needs of children and families.[8] Time is only one of several obstacles to providing the most effective care for behavioral health concerns. Pediatric providers typically have limited training in brief assessment and implementation of evidence-based psychosocial interventions for behavioral health concerns,[8,9] despite the role that they have in providing guidance to families. The result is that behavioral health needs of children in primary care may go unrecognized or interventions that might be beneficial are not offered.

There are several recommendations to reduce the behavioral health burden in primary care and increase access to evidence-based interventions for youth. One of the most promising is the integrated behavioral health model of service delivery.[3,10,11] In a fully integrated service, behavioral health clinicians are a part of the primary care team, work closely with providers and other team members (eg, nursing staff), share space and resources (eg, medical records), and provide same-day screenings, interventions, and/or consultations for patients.[3,10] These interventions typically are brief, time limited, and targeted toward a specific concern, in order to match the pace of primary care. Furthermore, the interventions often are pulled from current evidence-based psychosocial treatment packages, usually coming from behavioral and cognitive behavior approaches.[12,13] There is an emerging literature supporting the integrated behavioral health model in pediatric primary care, suggesting that it can increase access to behavioral health care, improve symptoms and quality of life, and promote greater patient satisfaction.[14–16] The potential to improve access to and delivery of behavioral health care has led to increased implementation in medical centers and community clinics.

Despite this potential, a vast majority of primary care providers still lack access to behavioral health clinicians in their practice.[17,18] There are many barriers to implementation, including health system constraints (eg, billing/financial) as well as workforce limitations (eg, training in interprofessional practice, attitudes toward team-based care, and understanding scopes of practice[19]). Until integration is widely adopted, pediatric providers may benefit from supplementing current methods of behavioral health management with strategies that behavioral health clinicians typically implement in integrated settings. Although less efficient than a warm hand-off to a behavioral health specialist, pediatric providers are well positioned to provide brief, action-oriented interventions in the context of health maintenance visits and acute visits.[20,21]

This article presents screening, brief intervention, and referral guidelines for the most prominent behavioral health problems seen in pediatric primary care: disruptive behavior disorders, attention-deficit/hyperactivity disorder (ADHD), anxiety disorders, depressive disorders, and substance use/abuse.[22,23] The structure of the clinical recommendations—screening, brief intervention, and referral to treatment as needed (SBIRT)—is based on an evidence-based approach to treating substance abuse in primary care[24] and provides a framework that easily is transferred to other problems seen in this setting. The screening measures selected for this review were chosen for their relative brevity, accessibility (ie, nonproprietary), and ease of administration and scoring, such that any provider might implement in a busy clinic as an augment to information gathered in interaction with the child and family (**Table 1**). Likewise, selection of the brief interventions was based on their simplicity of implementation and basis in empirically supported interventions that have shown some success with both majority youth and ethnic minority youth.[25] Lastly, guidelines are offered for when to refer to specialty mental health services, taking into account the American Academy of Pediatrics (AAP) practice recommendations.

Table 1
Behavioral health screening tools for pediatric primary care

Measure	Problem Area(s)	Age Range	Length and Format	Subscales	Cut-off Scores for Relevant Problem Area
NICHQ Vanderbilt	ADHD (primary), ODD, CD, anxiety, depression	6–12 y	55 items for parent report; 43 for teacher report; 26 items for both teacher and provider follow-up + medication side effects Rated on a never (0) to very often (3) scale for problem areas excellent (1) to problematic (5) for performance	ADHD (inattentive subtype, hyperactive/impulsivity subtype, and combined); ODD; CD; anxiety/depression; performance (academic and behavioral)	ADHD inattentive or ADHD hyperactive/impulsive: at least 6 positive responses (ie, score of 2 or 3) out of 9 questions on each respective subscale AND a score of 4 or 5 on any performance questions ADHD combined: requires the above criteria for both subscales ODD (parent): at least 4 positive responses out of 8 AND a score of 4 or 5 on any performance questions Conduct (parent): at least 3 positive responses out of 14 AND a score of 4 or 5 on any performance questions ODD/conduct (teacher): at least 3 positive responses out of 10 AND a score of 4 or 5 on any performance questions Anxiety/depression: at least 3 positive responses out of 7 AND a score of 4 or 5 on any performance questions

(continued on next page)

Table 1
(continued)

Measure	Problem Area(s)	Age Range	Length and Format	Subscales	Cut-off Scores for Relevant Problem Area
PSC-17	Attention, internalizing, and externalizing problems	4–16 y	17 items rated on a never (0), sometimes (1), or often (2) scale	Attention, internalizing (eg, anxiety and mood), and externalizing (eg, noncompliance and aggression)	Attention: ≥ 7 Internalizing: ≥ 5 Externalizing: ≥ 7 Total score: ≥ 15
SCARED for youth and parent	Anxiety	≥ 8 y	41 items rated on a not true or hardly ever true (0), somewhat true or sometimes true (1), or very true or often true (2) scale	Panic disorder or somatic symptoms; GAD; separation anxiety disorder; social anxiety disorder; school avoidance	Total score: ≥ 25 indicates probable anxiety disorder Panic/somatic: ≥ 7 indicates panic disorder or significant somatic symptoms GAD: ≥ 9 may indicate the disorder Separation anxiety disorder: ≥ 5 may indicate the disorder Social anxiety disorder: ≥ 8 may indicate the disorder School avoidance: ≥ 3 may indicate significant avoidance
GAD-2 GAD-7	Anxiety	11–17 y	2 or 7 items rated on a 0 (not at all) to 3 (nearly every day) scale	None	GAD-2: score ≥ 3 indicates possible anxiety disorder GAD-7: Mild symptoms: 5–9 (monitor) Moderate symptoms: 10–14 (possibly clinically significant condition; further assessment and or referral recommended) Severe symptoms: ≥ 15 (active treatment recommended)

PHQ-2 PHQ-9	Depression and suicidality	Adolescent	2 or 9 items rated on a 0 (not at all) to 3 (nearly every day) scale	None	PHQ-2: score $\geq$3 indicates possible depression PHQ-9: Minimal or no symptoms: 0–4 (monitor) Mild: 5–9 (use clinical judgment to determine treatment) Moderate: 10–14 (use clinical judgment to determine treatment) Moderately severe: 15–19 (warrants active treatment) Severe: 20–27 (warrants active treatment)
CES-DC	Depression	6–17 y	20 items rated on a not at all (0) to a lot (3) scale (some items reversed scored)	None	Score $\geq$15 significant symptoms of depression
S2BI	Substance use	Adolescents	7 items rating the frequency of use of several substances: never, once or twice, monthly, to weekly or more	None	Once or twice: low risk (unlikely to meet criteria for substance use disorder) Monthly: likely meet criteria for mild or moderate substance use disorder Weekly+: likely meet criteria for severe substance use disorder

(continued on next page)

Table 1
(continued)

Measure	Problem Area(s)	Age Range	Length and Format	Subscales	Cut-off Scores for Relevant Problem Area
BSTAD	Substance use	12–17 y	11 items for friend and personal use of substances as well as frequency of personal use	None	0 d: no reported use 1 d: lower risk 2+ d (alcohol or other drugs) and/or 6+ d (tobacco): higher risk

DISRUPTIVE BEHAVIOR DISORDERS

Disruptive behavior (eg, noncompliance or disobedience) is one of the most prominent issues seen in primary care.[26,27] At the severe end of the spectrum, disruptive behavior includes *Diagnostic and Statistical Manual of Mental Disorders* (Fifth Edition) *(DSM-5)* diagnoses, such as oppositional defiant disorder (ODD) and conduct disorder (CD), but most often involves subthreshold presentations or reactionary acting-out in response to transient events or stressors and/or as a part of developmental transitions. The common thread among disruptive behavior disorders is that behavior is directed outwardly toward others (ie, externalizing) and sometimes is considered a problem of under-control—children may be impulsive, oppositional, aggressive, and defiant of rules or authority.[28] What differentiates the disorders (from those who do not meet criteria for a diagnosis) is the severity, chronicity, and context in which the behavior is occurring. For instance, CD is characterized by violation of the rights of others via physical aggression or force as well as theft, deceitfulness, destruction of property, and serious violation of rules[29] and is a risk factor for antisocial personality disorder in adulthood. In contrast, ODD is characterized by angry/irritable mood, argumentative and noncompliant behavior, and vindictiveness.[29] Lifetime prevalence of CD is estimated at 9.5%[30] and of ODD is 10.2%.[31] Previous estimates have suggested that approximately 3.5% of children currently exhibit behavioral or conduct problems.[32,33]

Screening

The AAP Task Force on Mental Health (TFOMH) has provided guidelines for the screening of behavioral and emotional concerns across all age groups at well-child visits and/or if problems are observed during a visit, psychosocial changes have occurred, or concerns are reported.[21,34] Although a majority of disruptive behavior measures are proprietary in nature and lengthy, two measures commonly used in primary care can serve as screeners and even aid in diagnosis (see **Table 1**). The National Institute for Children's Health Quality (NICHQ) Vanderbilt Assessment Scale is typically used in the assessment of ADHD and offers subscales for CD and ODD (separately for parent report and combined for the teacher report), given their comorbidity with ADHD.[35] Second, the Pediatric Symptom Checklist (PSC)-17 is a broad psychosocial screening measure and includes an externalizing behavior subscale.[36,37]

Brief Intervention

Regardless of diagnosis or severity, children displaying disruptive behaviors can benefit from behavioral interventions that seek to increase positive alternatives and decrease undesirable responding. Most evidence-based treatments for childhood disruptive behaviors involve teaching caregivers how to influence behavior, particularly using principles of operant learning.[38–41] A recommended method for decreasing undesirable behavior (eg, noncompliance or teasing) is to identify and intentionally reinforce its positive opposite (eg, minding and cooperating). Reinforcing (immediately and consistently) behaviors one wants to increase is a generalizable strategy for many presenting problems and is foundational for behavior change interventions. Focusing on reinforcing positive opposites, before using disciplinary strategies, also helps improve strained caregiver-child relations. **Box 1** presents strategies for using reinforcement to improve desired behavior and recommended steps when implementing a formal incentive system. Age and developmental factors are important to keep in mind with these strategies. Younger children often need more frequent and immediate reinforcement, and what serves as a reinforcer varies with age. Token systems can be

---

Box 1
How to use reinforcement to influence child behavior[38,39]

1. Choose behaviors to reinforce. Specify exactly what those behaviors look or sound like (so that even a stranger could identify occurrences), such as getting dressed, keeping hands to oneself, looking at parent when being spoken to, and so forth.
   - Tip: make clear to the child what the expectations are and that the child has the skills to do the requested behavior.

2. Create opportunities for the child to engage in the behavior and "catch them being good."
   - Tip: when creating an opportunity, at a suitable time, give a direct command in a neutral voice ("Please clean your room now."), and, if possible, include reference to a benefit to the child ("We'll then have extra family movie time later.")

3. Immediately praise when the child engages in desired behavior.
   - Tip: praise frequently and enthusiastically. Specify what the child did well ("Thanks for starting right away when I asked you." or "You're getting good at making the bed.") and supplement with hugs, smiles, high fives, nods, and winks, and so forth, as developmentally appropriate.

4. Use a formal incentive system to supplement the use of praise.
   - Tips for a successful rewards system:
     o Specify 1–5 behaviors that will earn tokens.
     o Select something to serve as tokens (points, stickers, check marks, marbles, poker chips, or clothes pins).
     o Assign a value for each specified behavior in token units.
     o Consistently award tokens immediately after behavior occurs.
     o Track earnings (on a chart or in a jar).
     o Develop a reward menu for child to cash in tokens.

---

faded out once improvement in child behavior stabilizes. The use of labeled praise (ie, verbally telling children precisely what they did that was liked) and other immediate positive social consequences for desired behavior (eg, high fives, knuckle knocks, hugs, accolades, and statements of pride) are recommended as a general parenting strategy that can be used frequently regardless of age or situation.[38–41]

Referral

There are no AAP guidelines for diagnosis and treatment of disruptive behavior disorders in children. Referral to specialty treatment involves a clinical judgment of severity of problem behavior (informed by the assessment devices recommended in **Table 1**), family capacities, and caregiver preferences. Parent training is the treatment of choice for children with disruptive behavior diagnoses[42,43] and can be useful for children with subthreshold problems as a prevention strategy.[40] In outpatient mental health settings, a course of parent training typically is delivered in 10 sessions to 20 sessions, although it has been adapted for delivery in primary care.[44] For adolescents, adding individual cognitive behavior therapy (CBT) or multisystemic therapy can augment changes in caregiving practices.[42]

ATTENTION-DEFICIT/HYPERACTIVITY DISORDER

ADHD is one of the most prevalent of childhood disorders frequently managed in primary care.[33,45] Children diagnosed with ADHD exhibit difficulty sustaining attention to tasks, difficulty inhibiting behavior or controlling impulses, and/or hyperactivity that begins before age 12, is not developmentally normative, and causes impairment in more than one setting.[29] These primary symptom clusters allow diagnosticians to specify whether a child presents with combined inattention/hyperactivity, predominately inattentive, or predominately hyperactive/impulsive symptoms.[29] A national survey in 2016 found a lifetime prevalence of 9.4%, with 8.4% reporting as current cases and higher rates in boys than girls.[46] Comorbidity is the norm with ADHD, with more than two-thirds of children also experiencing one other co-occurring condition (most often disruptive behavior disorders[46]). The AAP considers ADHD a chronic condition that requires ongoing management through childhood.[47]

Screening

The AAP recommends ADHD screening for children ages 4 to 18 who are experiencing behavioral or academic problems and any of the 3 symptom clusters.[47] The most widely used screening measure for ADHD in primary care is the NICHQ Vanderbilt,[35] which has 2 specific subscales for ADHD (inattention and hyperactive/impulsive) that correspond directly with DSM-5 criteria (see **Table 1**). The Vanderbilt also provides subscales for comorbid conditions (eg, ODD/conduct and anxiety/depression). Differential diagnosis is important to identify whether children are presenting with ADHD and comorbid disruptive behavior or if the presenting problem is better characterized by disruptive behavior only. A positive ADHD screen can inform decision making about whether to pursue a multimethod, multi-informant assessment to confirm the diagnosis. The PSC-17 also provides an attention subscale in addition to externalizing behavior.[36,37] Although less comprehensive, positive scores on the attention subscale could alert clinicians to potential ADHD problems and suggest follow-up or intervention.

Brief Intervention

Although stimulant medications and nonstimulant alternatives are widely prescribed in pediatric primary care and are recommended as treatment of ADHD in children ages 6 and up,[47] behavioral interventions also have shown promise in the treatment of ADHD either alone[43,48] and/or in conjunction with medications.[49,50] For children under age 6, behavioral interventions are the first-line treatment of ADHD.[47] Given estimates that less than half of children with a current ADHD diagnosis have received behavioral treatment in the past year,[46] providing behavioral interventions in primary care may have additive benefit. Similar to disruptive behavior disorders, evidence-based psychosocial interventions for ADHD are based on operant learning theory and often use parent training as a key component.[48] Considering ADHD as a disorder of self-regulation, interventions that focus both on externalizing antecedents (specifically, prompts, which directly facilitate performance of a behavior) and consequences (ie, reinforcers) are particularly important.[51] Children with ADHD often need more specific prompts (signs, lists, cards, charts, or posters) and consistent structure/routine to help them stay on task; they also benefit from immediate, frequent, and meaningful consequences for following through with those tasks.[52] Given that children with ADHD exhibit problems in school—academic, social, and behavioral—one simple yet effective intervention is a daily school–home report card.[52,53]

Box 2 highlights the key strategies in implementing a daily school–home report card. This method facilitates management of behavior in multiple settings (school and home) by linking rewards at home to behavior during the school day. The report card specifies and prompts target behaviors in the classroom and encourages regular feedback from the teacher, which can bridge the gap until delivery of a tangible reward at home. It also serves as a communication tool between teachers and caregivers and ideally facilitates consistent responding to child behavior by multiple individuals.

Box 2
How to set up a daily school–home report card[52,53]

1. In conjunction with child's teacher and/or school staff, select behaviors to target.
   - Tips for selecting and defining behaviors:
     - In children with ADHD, academic work (eg, staying on task), peer relations (eg, taking turns), and rule-following all are potentially important targets.
     - Specify behaviors that can be observed and counted throughout the day. Examples: plays without fighting, completes and returns homework, obeys teacher when command is given
     - Choose 3–5 behaviors to start.

2. Select target criteria for each behavior based on how frequently behavior currently is occurring, while taking into account different class periods.
   - Tip: choose achievable goal and modify as the child progresses. Example: fewer than 2 interruptions during each class period

3. Develop a tracking form
   - Tip: add rewards for successfully bringing tracking form to school and back home.

4. Create or supplement a home-based rewards system (see **Box 1**). Children should have access to a menu of daily and weekly rewards created with their input.
   - Tip: make fewer or less preferred rewards earned by less positive remarks and more larger or salient rewards contingent on better performance.

5. Monitor progress and troubleshoot as needed. Make criteria more challenging as child exhibits improved performance in behavior.
   - Tip: consider all aspects of the plan before terminating or implementing alternative options. Some questions to ask: Are the target behaviors appropriate? Is the teacher able to monitor the child's behavior? Is the child receiving sufficient feedback? Are the rewards motivating? Are the rewards being delivered consistently?

Example School–Home Report Card

Target Behaviors	Subject 1	Subject 2	Lunch	Recess	Subject 3	Subject 4	Subject 5
1. Turned in assignments appropriately	Y N	Y N	Y N	Y N	Y N	Y N	Y N
2. Followed rules with ≤2 violations	Y N	Y N	Y N	Y N	Y N	Y N	Y N
3. Bothered others during seat work ≤2 times	Y N	Y N	Y N	Y N	Y N	Y N	Y N
4. Raised hand to speak with ≤2 violations	Y N	Y N	Y N	Y N	Y N	Y N	Y N
5. Other _____	Y N	Y N	Y N	Y N	Y N	Y N	Y N

Tally the "yeses" and "nos" and deliver back-up reinforcers accoding to plan
Rule of thumb: Initially twice the "yeses" to "nos" is considered a successful day

---

One facet of academic underperformance in ADHD is problems with homework completion. Battles over homework can lead to negative caregiver-child interactions and incompletion impairs learning and results in lower grades. **Box 3** provides recommendations for teaching caregivers how to implement homework sessions in a way that can naturally complement other incentive systems (see **Boxes 1–2**).

Referral

Although medication management can be handled in the primary care medical home, other recommended interventions for ADHD generally require involvement with a mental health professional or the educational system. Per AAP recommendations,[47]

Box 3
How to set up a daily homework session[51]

1. Break homework into 15–20-minute sessions with 5-minute breaks in-between.
   • Expand or contract the times based on age and individual differences.

2. Create a conducive study environment for homework sessions.
   • Distraction-free (quiet or with some ambient background noise or music)
   • Sitting upright
   • Flat surface
   • Well lit

3. Establish a routine time for homework sessions to begin.

4. Prior to study session, have the child
   • Exercise for 10–15 minutes (take a brief walk or bike ride, stretch or do calisthenics, or shoot baskets).
   • Practice mediation or relaxation breathing (exhales longer than inhales) for several minutes.
   • Collaborate to identify a reasonable outcome goal for the session.

5. During the study session
   Have the child intermittently
   • Visualize the outcome and reward for completing work.
   • Rehearse self-affirming and encouraging statements.
   • Consume a glucose-rich beverage (sports drink or lemonade).
   Have the caregiver
   • Oversee the session.
   • Provide prompts and reinforcement for goal-directed behavior.
   • Assist as needed.

---

school-aged children and adolescents with ADHD incrementally benefit from parent management training and/or behavioral classroom interventions as well as educational support (eg, an individualized education plan). Although primary care clinicians can get the ball rolling on behavior management by introducing the daily school–home report card (or a similar intervention), some children and families may need more assistance in planning and implementing behavior management plans. These more comprehensive services, including comprehensive diagnostic evaluations, typically require coordination between an outpatient mental health provider and the school system.

ANXIETY DISORDERS

Excessive fear and anxious arousal, disproportionate apprehension, and life-interfering avoidance behavior characterize anxiety disorders in children. There is much overlap in terms of symptom/behavioral presentation and significant comorbidity. As such, what differentiates each diagnosis is determined by identifying the types of situations the child avoids and that produce anxiety and fear and the thoughts/beliefs about the danger faced in those situations. Common anxieties (and the related anxiety disorders) in children include the following: being away from, and harm befalling, caregivers (separation anxiety disorder); heights, snakes, insects, injections (specific phobias); social scrutiny or evaluation (social anxiety disorder); uncertainty about competence, school, or friendships (generalized anxiety disorder [GAD]); heightened sensitivity to physiologic sensations (panic disorder); confronting reminders of negative events (posttraumatic stress disorder [PTSD]); and unwanted thoughts or urges (obsessive compulsive disorder [OCD][29]). The *DSM-5* placed PTSD and OCD in chapters separate from anxiety disorders.[29] They are included in this article because they share characteristics with anxiety disorders and can benefit from similar treatment approaches. Anxiety disorders often start in early childhood.[54] Point prevalence estimates suggest that approximately 3% of children ages 4 to 17 experience current anxiety problems.[32,33] Lifetime estimates in adolescents suggest approximately 1 in 3 experiences an anxiety disorder, with specific phobia the most frequently reported (approximately 20%), followed by social anxiety disorder (9.1%), and separation anxiety disorder (76%).[54] Anxiety and avoidance are fundamentally adaptive responses to perceived threat, and many fears are developmentally appropriate at certain ages/stages. Anxiety becomes clinically relevant when it is excessive, persistent, and interferes with daily functioning and a child's ability to participate in age-appropriate social and educational activities.

Screening

Although there are no AAP specific guidelines for the screening of anxiety disorders, the TFOMH suggests general screening of emotional and behavioral problems across the life span if problems are observed during a visit, psychosocial changes have occurred, or concerns are reported.[21,34] As outlined in **Table 1**, the Screen for Childhood Anxiety Related Emotional Disorders (SCARED) is a relatively brief measure of youth anxiety (excluding OCD or PTSD), for children ages 8 and up.[55] It has both parent and youth versions and provides a total score that can indicate a probable anxiety problem. For adolescents specifically, the GAD 2-item and 7-item scales assess experiences with anxiety symptoms over the prior 2 weeks.[56] Lastly, the broad-based PSC-17 also has an internalizing subscale, although a majority of items are related to mood (cutoff: 5 or above[36,37]). During screening, it is important to differentiate between persistent life-altering anxieties (lasting months) versus transient anxieties due to environmental stressors (eg, starting a new school).

Brief Intervention

Anxiety disorders share a similar underlying psychological process—the experience of anxiety or fear physiologically (eg, heart palpitations or sweating), anxious thinking (eg, expecting the worse to occur), and behavioral escape (eg, leave situation) or avoidance (eg, avoid situation[57]). Escape and avoidance of fear/anxiety-provoking situations is the primary mechanism maintaining problematic anxiety. Escape and avoidance temporally reduce/eliminate anxious arousal, thus strengthening (via negative reinforcement) these behaviors while also solidifying associated exaggerated interpretations of anxious arousal and the likelihood of negative outcomes. As such, intervention includes strategies to help youth understand anxious arousal as an uncomfortable but nondangerous well-characterized bodily response (psychoeducation), interpret anxiety-evoking situations as an opportunity for coping skill use (cognitive flexibility), and behave in the face of anxiety to learn they can cope and experience previously avoided contexts in a new way (exposure to feared stimuli).[57–61]

Box 4 highlights practical steps for teaching children to cope with anxiety adapted from a cognitive behavioral treatment of childhood and adolescent anxiety with demonstrated efficacy.[61–63] The 4 main components are (1) identifying experiences of anxiety and when they occur; (2) learning strategies for responding to anxious physiologic arousa; (3) identifying and responding in new ways to anxious thinking; and (4) creating a plan for learning and practicing how to cope with the experience of anxiety without escaping or avoiding the situation. It is important to create a coping plan that emphasizes gradual exposure to anxiety-provoking objects, events, or situations. Exposure to feared stimuli, where negative expectations are not fully realized, appears

---

Box 4
How to teach children to cope with anxiety

1. Help children identify anxious feelings in the body and the situations in which those anxious feelings occur.
   - Tips for identification:
     - Provide psychoeducation on how anxiety and fear are felt physically and model where people typically feel anxiety/fear (eg, upset stomach).
     - Teach children to rate feelings of anxiety/fear on a 1–10 scale and the situations in which they occur.

2. Teach child relaxation strategies
   - Courage breath
     - Lift shoulders toward ears on inhalation, rotate back (bringing shoulder blades together) as exhalation starts, and return down as exhalation finishes.
   - Tense and release
     - Inhale and flex (for several seconds) and then exhale and release various muscle groups to identify bodily sensations of tension and relaxation.
   - Belly breathing
     - With 1 hand on stomach and the other on chest
     - Breath in deep through nose, pushing hand on belly out, while chest does not move.
     - Breathe out slowly through mouth, feeling hand on belly go in.

3. Teach children to identify and respond back to anxious thinking.
   - Questions for identification: "What are you expecting to occur?" and "What is your self-talk?"
   - Questions for challenging: "Do you know for sure this may happen?" "How likely is that to happen?" and "What is the worst that can occur?"

4. Teach children to cope effectively in the presence of anxiety provoking situations.
   - Tip for coping with thoughts:
     - Encourage children to come up with coping thoughts ("What is a different way to think about this?" and "What would you tell a friend to think or do?")
   - Tips for coping with behavior:
     - Encourage children to approach feared situations gradually using a coping model ("What small step can you take to cope differently in this situation?" and "How can you stay in that situation even when you feel anxious?").
     - Provide praise and rewards for effort and progress.

---

critical for new learning (and hence improvement) to occur.[58,64] Gradual exposure involves working with youth and families to implement small steps to approaching feared situations. For instance, a child who is fearful of sleeping alone at night first may sleep with a parent in the room and then may sleep with a parent in the room part of the night, gradually moving up to where the parent no longer is in the bedroom and the child no longer needs the parent's presence to fall asleep. Moving to the next phase of exposure follows successful completion of previous exposures, characterized often by decreased anxiety and increased mastery of coping in the identified situation.

Referral

There are no AAP guidelines for diagnosis and treatment of anxiety disorders, so the basis for referral is clinical judgment of severity and the needs and wants of the family. An 8-session to 12-session behavioral intervention for anxiety and depression, which approximates mental health specialty care but was delivered in a primary care setting, has demonstrated efficacy.[65,66] In the absence of behavioral health specialists embedded in the primary care clinic, consideration of referral to mental health specialty care appears warranted for any probable anxiety disorder diagnosis, with CBT the recommended first-line intervention.[59,60] Medication management is another option. Both CBT and sertraline outperform a pill placebo for children with diagnosed anxiety and related disorders, with the combination resulting in the highest response rates.[67–69]

DEPRESSIVE DISORDERS

Many youth experience depression or depressive symptoms, often characterized by low mood and/or irritability, lack of interest or pleasure in activities, and several physical (eg, low energy, sleep problems, and fatigue) and cognitive (eg, difficulty concentrating, low self-esteem, and suicidal ideation) symptoms.[29] Younger children are less likely to report significant depressive symptoms[54,70]; however, prevalence rates increase during adolescence.[54,71] The 12-month prevalence of major depressive disorder or dysthymia in adolescents (ages 13–17) is approximately 8.2% and any mood disorder diagnosis is approximately 10%.[71] Lifetime prevalence is approximately 12% for major depressive disorder or dysthymia and approximately 14% for all mood disorders, with girls more likely to report symptoms.[54] Mood disorders often are recurrent, with many individuals who experience depression in adolescence also often experiencing additional episodes during their life course.[72]

Screening

The AAP suggests all children ages 12 and older should be screened for depression annually and children at high risk for depression (eg, parent history of depression, substance use, or suicidal ideation) should be targeted and assessed more frequently during preventative and health care visits.[73] **Table 1** outlines the most prominent screeners for depression in primary care, which are the patient health questionnaire (PHQ)-2[74] and PHQ-9.[75] The PHQ-2 asks about experiences of the 2 cardinal symptoms of depression—low mood and little interest or pleasure in doing things—during the past week, whereas the PHQ-9 asks all of the questions contained in the *DSM-5* criteria for a major depressive episode. Another freely available measure that is more specific to younger children (ages 6–17) is the Center for Epidemiological Studies Depression Scale modified for children and adolescents (CES-DC).[76] Lastly, as discussed previously, the broad band measure PSC-17 has an internalizing subscale related to mood symptoms.

Brief Intervention

Depression is characterized by passive/avoidant behaviors (eg, isolation), often precipitated by environmental changes or stressors, and which contribute to low mood and negative thinking.[77,78] This passive/avoidant behavior is considered the key mechanism in maintaining and worsening depression and is a straightforward target for intervention.[77–79] Behavioral activation (BA) has emerged as an evidence-based treatment of depression[80] and seeks to reduce passive behavioral patterns and increase engagement in activities that are pleasant, valued, and social and increase feelings of mastery.[81] Individuals are aided in planning activities that are likely to be positively reinforcing. This engagement has a secondary effect of improving low mood and other symptoms. Implementation with adolescents shows promise.[82–86] Importantly, the simple idea of getting active when feeling down makes it an easy intervention to implement in primary care.

Despite its relative ease to implement, BA can be challenging for patients to do. **Box 5** outlines steps to take when planning activity scheduling with children and adolescents. The use of an activity planner (**Fig. 1**) is recommended to help youth think

---

Box 5
Activity scheduling

1. Goal is to behave based on a plan, not on mood.
   - Adaptive strategy —when facing obstacles and feeling down, stay active.
     - Benefit is having more control over behavior and, because actions link to thoughts and feelings, can lead to beneficial spirals (eg, see a friend, realize you are cared about, and feel better).

   Rather than
   - Passive strategy—wait until you feel better, more motivated, etc. to get active.
     - Problem is you have less direct control over mood and, because mood links to actions and thoughts, can lead to depressive spirals (eg, feel down, stay at home, and thinking you are a loser).

2. Brainstorm a list of potential activities the child can schedule over the next week. Choose a range of activities to try and hit the following targets:
   - Experiences as pleasurable (eg, riding a bike)
   - Provides a sense of mastery (eg, finishing a puzzle or shooting lay-ups)
   - Involves others (eg, interactions with peers, siblings, or caregivers)
   - Relate to values, that is, what is important and inherently reinforcing to child (eg, spending time with family)
   - Tip: as a starting point, identify activities the child already may be engaging in to some extent or that were enjoyed previously.

3. Schedule activities to occur throughout the week. Start small, with goals that are achievable and realistic, that the child agrees can be done regardless of mood. Have the child monitor mood while engaging in activities.
   - Tip: encourage children to notice relationships between behavior and mood for 2 purposes:
     - To show child that s/he can activate, to some extent, independent of mood
       1. Promotes sense of agency
     - To learn what activities or events lead to better mood
       1. Promotes self-understanding and planning—How can we plan more of these activities? When feeling low, what actions can one take to get out of it?

---

ahead about when the activities can and will occur and to monitor mood and its relationship with behavior. An important component of activity scheduling is teaching children to take action based on a plan, rather than on their feelings. Having a tangible written plan makes that point concrete. After gaining traction, children experientially learn that mood states and negative thinking tend to improve along with behavior change, and formal scheduling of activities can be faded out.

Referral

The AAP provides specific guidance on treatment recommendations.[87] Mild depression requires only active support and monitoring for approximately 6 weeks to 8 weeks. Persistent symptoms (after 6–8 weeks), moderate or severe symptoms, and/or complicating factors warrant consultation with a mental health specialist. As discussed previously, 8 sessions to 12 sessions of CBT delivered in a primary care setting demonstrated efficacy,[65,66] and another recommended treatment—pharmacotherapy with selective serotonin reuptake inhibitors (SSRIs)—is readily available in primary care. Brief CBT in conjunction with medications also have demonstrated preliminary effectiveness in primary care.[88,89] If referring to mental health specialty care, recommended treatments include CBT (including BA) or interpersonal psychotherapy for adolescents.[87] A standard course of care is 10 sessions to 20 sessions but might be longer if treatment is continued until 6 months of symptom remission is achieved. A

ACTION PLAN	Morning	Completed	Mood	Afternoon	Completed	Mood	Evening	Completed	Mood
Day	Scheduled activities	Y/N	1-10	Scheduled activities	Y/N	1-10	Scheduled activities	Y/N	1-10
Sunday	Read inspirational scripture passages			Play a card game with sister			Popcorn and watch singing show with family		
	Send a positive text to a friend			Take dog for a walk			Bath & read to relax before bed		
Monday									
Tuesday									
Wednesday									
Thursday									
Friday									
Saturday									

A mood rating of 1 is equivalent to the worse mood of your entire life and 10 is the most positive mood ever experienced in your life.

For illustrative purposes, some representative activities were entered for Sunday.

Fig. 1. Activity scheduling weekly planner.

combination of CBT and SSRIs appears to accelerate treatment response in moderate to severe cases, although, after several months, monotherapies were just as effective as combination treatment (with CBT having less adverse events than medications[90–92]).

SUBSTANCE USE DISORDER

Alcohol and illicit drug use in youth has been decreasing over the past few decades.[23] There still are, however, a substantial proportion of youth using substances and a smaller minority who meet criteria for substance use disorder,[93] characterized by use that leads to significant impairment and failure to meet major life responsibilities.[29] In 2018, an estimated 1.6% of adolescents (ages 12–17) met criteria for an alcohol use disorder, whereas 2.7% met criteria for an illicit drug use disorder and 2.1% for marijuana use disorder.[93] Lifetime prevalence for any substance use disorder is approximately 11%.[54] When it comes to drug use in general, approximately 1 in 11 adolescents was considered a current alcohol user, contrasted with 1 in 6 illicit drug users and 1 in 8 marijuana users.[93] Many youth who engage in substance use often meet criteria for other co-occurring mental health conditions.

Screening

The AAP provides specific guidelines for SBIRT for adolescent substance use.[94,95] All adolescents should be screened for substance use at health maintenance visits and/ or when circumstances may suggest potential substance use (eg, decline in grades).[34] The Screening to Brief Intervention (S2BI) tool screens for all use of substances and frequency, providing risk categories that can help guide intervention.[96] The Brief Screener for Tobacco, Alcohol, and Other Drugs (BSTAD) asks how frequently teens use alcohol, tobacco, and marijuana over the past year[97] and also gives risk ratings based on frequency of use.

Brief Intervention

After identifying a youth with moderate risk to high risk for a substance use disorder (or risky use without meeting criteria for a disorder), the AAP generally recommends having a dialogue with patients that encourages healthy choices and attempts to reduce risky behaviors.[95] When youth show defensiveness or resistance to direct recommendations, one style of dialogue is motivational interviewing (MI).[98,99] MI is an evidence-based approach that focuses on strengthening motivation to change, while respecting patient autonomy. As opposed to specific techniques or strategies, MI is a way of having a productive conversation about a potential problem that reduces resistance and helps patients clarify their perspective, a precursor to deciding what changes (if any) to make. One of the most prominent MI skills is open-ended questions, affirmations, reflections, and summaries (OARS).[98,99]

Table 2 defines each OARS skill and includes examples of questions or statements a clinician might make. What makes MI a client-centered but also directive approach is a practitioner's differential attending to change talk. As the conversation progresses, the practitioner asks more open-ended questions linked to prior patient change talk, and affirms, reflects, and summarizes with differential emphasis on the youth's change talk. The important component of this unique style is that as opposed to lecturing the patient and providing reasons to stop using, the MI practitioner listens to the youth, asks nonjudgmentally about substance use (and its impact), and uses that information to help the individual consider seriously the prospect of change. **Box 6** shows a specific MI technique referred to as the decisional balance.

Table 2		
Motivational interviewing open-ended questions, affirmations, reflections, and summaries skill description and examples		
Skill	**Description/Function**	**Examples**
Open-ended questions	Frames a question that requires an explanation and/or elaboration. Requires the patient to elaborate on change talk; can help clinician and patient formulate a change plan	"What are some reasons you have considered cutting down on drinking?" "What are some barriers to you making that change?"
Affirmations	Validates behavior change, strengths, and abilities, and/or autonomy. Reinforces change talk	"You've spent a lot of time thinking about how drinking impacts you." "It sounds like you know what is best for you."
Reflections	Demonstrates listening and empathy. Can be a method of "rolling with resistance" to change or reinforcing change talk	"You aren't sure if you're ready to quit drinking." "Quitting would make you feel better physically."
Summaries	Connecting the dots of a conversation; providing a description of what was spoken about. Incorporating and ending with motivating statements	"You've told me a lot about why you have been drinking—it relaxes you and you have fun when you are with your friends. At the same time, you're worried about how it may affect your health and what would happen if your parents found out. You are not sure about quitting, and are still worried about the consequences."

Box 6
Decisional balance—a strategy for assessing and possibly enhancing motivation to change

1. In a decisional balance discussion, a youth identified as engaging in risky substance use is asked to respond to open-ended questions about
   - The pros of the current pattern of use
   - The cons of changing the current pattern of use
   - The cons of the current pattern of use
   - The pros of changing the current pattern of use

Tip: key to using the decisional balance in an MI consistent fashion is placing a greater emphasis on reflecting and asking follow-up questions about the pros of changing and the cons of the status quo.

2. The decisional balance also can be completed collaboratively as, or transcribed onto, a sheet.

Target behavior: _____

	Pros / Benefits	Cons / Costs
Status quo	Step 1	Step 3
Change	Step 4	Step 2

Referral

Referral typically is suggested for moderate cases that do not improve after a brief intervention and for all severe cases.[95] These instances likely necessitate the more intensive services of a mental health specialist or substance use specialist. Depending on the substances used and the regularity of use, severe cases may require partial hospitalization or residential treatment.

SUMMARY

Behavioral health problems routinely present in primary care. Primary care providers are generalists working in a fast-paced world. The need for brief screeners and straightforward interventions is apparent if behavioral health is to be addressed in this setting, especially in clinics that do not have fully integrated behavioral health specialists. This article provides examples of brief assessments and interventions for common presenting problems: disruptive behavior, ADHD, anxiety, depression, and substance misuse. The strategies were culled from empirically supported treatments and tailored for use in primary care. The authors hope they are helpful to pediatric providers seeking to augment their behavioral health management skill set and as a starting point for behavioral health providers embedded in primary care.

REFERENCES

1. Kessler R, Stafford D. Primary care *is* the de facto mental health system. In: Kessler R, Stafford D, editors. Collaborative medicine case studies: evidence in practice. New York, NY: Springer; 2008. p. 9–21.
2. Norquist GS, Regier DA. The epidemiology of psychiatric disorders and the de facto mental health care system. Annu Rev Med 1996;47:473–9.
3. Robinson PJ, Reiter JT. Behavioral health consultation and primary care: a guide to integrating services. second edition. New York, NY: Springer; 2016.
4. Costello EJ. Primary care pediatrics and child psychopathology: a review of diagnostic, treatment, and referral practices. Pediatrics 1986;78(6):1044–51.
5. Rushton J, Bruckman D, Kelleher K. Primary care referral of children with psychosocial problems. Arch Pediatr Adolesc Med 2002;156(6):592–8.
6. Kelleher KJ, Hohmann AA, Larson DB. Prescription of psychotropics to children in office-based practice. Am J Dis Child 1989;143(7):855–9.
7. Mark TL, Levit KR, Buck JA. Datapoints: psychotropic drug prescriptions by medical specialty. Psychiatr Serv 2009;60(9):1167.
8. Horwitz SM, Storfer-Isser A, Kerker BD, et al. Barriers to the identification and management of psychosocial problems: changes from 2004 to 2013. Acad Pediatr 2015;15(6):613–20.
9. Petts R, Shahidullah JD, Kettlewell PK, et al. As a pediatrician, I don't know the second, third, or fourth thing to do: a qualitative study of pediatric residents' training and experiences in behavioral health. Int J Health Sci Educ 2018;5(1). Available at: https://dc.etsu.edu/ijhse/vol5/iss1/5.
10. Reiter JT, Dobmeyer AC, Hunter CL. The primary care behavioral health (PCBH) model: an overview and operational definition. J Clin Psychol Med Settings 2018;25(2):109–26.
11. Kolko DJ, Perrin EC. The integration of behavioral health interventions in children's health care: services, sciences, and suggestions. J Clin Child Adolesc Psychol 2014;43(2):216–28.
12. Bridges AJ, Gregus SJ, Rodriguez JH, et al. Diagnoses, intervention strategies, and rates of functional improvement in integrated behavioral health care patients. J Consult Clin Psychol 2015;83(3):590–601.
13. Hunter CL, Goodie JL, Oordt MS, et al. Integrating behavioral health in primary care: step-by-step guidance for assessment and intervention. second edition. Washington, DC: American Psychological Association; 2009.
14. Asarnow JR, Rozenman M, Wiblin J, et al. Integrated medical-behavioral care compared with usual primary care for child and adolescent behavioral health: a meta-analysis. JAMA Pediatr 2015;169(10):929–37.
15. Burkhart K, Asogwa K, Muzaffar N, et al. Pediatric integrated care models: a systematic review. Clin Pediatr 2020;59(2):148–53.
16. Yonek J, Lee CM, Harrison A, et al. Key components of effective pediatric integrated mental health care models: a systematic review. JAMA Pediatr 2020;174(5):487–98.
17. Miller BF, Petterson S, Brown Levey SM, et al. Primary care, behavioral health, provider colocation and rurality. J Am Board Fam Med 2014;27(3):367–74.
18. Richman EL, Lombardi BM, Zerden LDS, et al. Where is behavioral health integration occurring? Mapping national co-location trends using national provider identifier data. Ann Arbor, MI: Behavioral health workforce Research center, University of Michigan; 2018. Available at: http://www.behavioralhealthworkforce.org/wp-content/uploads/2018/12/NPI-Full-Report_Final.pdf. Accessed July 24, 2020.

19. Wakida EK, Talib ZM, Akena D, et al. Barriers and facilitators to the integration of mental health services into primary health care: a systematic review. Syst Rev 2018;7:211.

20. Glascoe FP, Trimm F. Brief approaches to developmental-behavioral promotion in primary care: updates on methods and technology. Pediatrics 2014;133(5):884–97.

21. Foy JM, Kelleher KJ, Laraque D. Enhancing pediatric mental health care: strategies for preparing a primary care practice. Pediatrics 2010;125(3):S87–108.

22. Cassidy LJ, Jellinek MS. Approaches to recognition and management of childhood psychiatric disorders in pediatric primary care. J Child Adolesc Psychopharmacol 1998;45(5):1037–52.

23. Centers for Disease Control and Prevention. Mental health surveillance among children – United States, 2005-2011. Morbidity Mortality Weekly Rep 2013;62(Suppl2):1–35.

24. Agerwala SM, McCance-Katz EF. Integrating screening, brief intervention, and referral to treatment (SBIRT) into clinical practice settings: a brief review. J Psychoactive Drugs 2012;44(4):307–17.

25. Holly LE, Pina AA. Evidence-based treatments for mental, emotional, and behavioral problems in ethnic minority children and adolescents. In: Alfano CA, Beidel ED, editors. Comprehensive evidence based interventions for children and adolescents. Hoboken, NJ: John Wiley & Sons, Inc; 2014. p. 43–54.

26. Weitzman CC, Leventhal JM. Screening for behavioral health problems in primary care. Curr Opin Pediatr 2006;18(6):641–8.

27. Briggs-Gowan MJ, Horwitz SM, Schwab-Stone ME, et al. Mental health in pediatric settings: distribution of disorders and factors related to service use. J Am Acad Child Adolesc Psychiatry 2000;39(7):841–9.

28. Liu J. Childhood externalizing behavior: theory and implications. J Child Adolesc Psychiatr Nurs 2004;17(3):93–103.

29. American Psychiatric Association. Diagnostic and statistical manual of mental disorders. Fiveth edition. Washington, DC: Author; 2013.

30. Nock MK, Kazdin AE, Hiripi E, et al. Prevalence, subtypes, and correlates of DSM-IV conduct disorder in the national comorbidity survey replication. Psychol Med 2006;36:699–710.

31. Nock MK, Kazdin AE, Hiripi E, et al. Lifetime prevalence, correlates, and persistence of oppositional defiant disorder: results from the national comorbidity survey replication. J Child Psychol Psychiatry 2007;48(7):703–13.

32. Blumberg SJ, Foster EB, Frasier AM, et al. Design and operation of the national survey of Children's health, 2007. Hyattsville, MD: National Center for Health Statistics; 2009.

33. Perou R, Bitsko RH, Blumberg SJ, et al, Centers for Disease Control and Prevention (CDC). Mental health surveillance among children: United States, 2005–2011. MMWR Surveill Summ 2013;62(suppl 2):1–35.

34. American Academy of Pediatrics. Appendix S4: the case for routine mental health screening. Pediatrics 2010;125(suppl 3):S133–9.

35. Wolraich ML, Lambert W, Doffing MA, et al. Psychometric properties of the Vanderbilt ADHD diagnostic parent rating scale in a referred population. J Pediatr Psychol 2003;28:559–67.

36. Jellinek MS, Murphy JM, Little M, et al. Use of the Pediatric Symptom Checklist to screen for psychosocial problems in pediatric primary care: a national feasibility study. Arch Pediatr Adolesc Med 1999;153:254–60.

37. Gardner W, Lucas A, Kolko DJ, et al. Comparison of the PSC-17 and alternative mental health screens in an at-risk primary care sample. J Am Acad Child Adolesc Psychiatry 2007;46:611–8.

38. Weiz JR, Kazdin AE. Evidence-based psychotherapies for children and adolescents. New York: Guilford Press; 2010.

39. Kazdin AE. Parent management training: treatment for oppositional, aggressive, and antisocial behavior in children and adolescents. New York, NY: Oxford University Press; 2005.

40. Leijten P, Gardner F, Melendez-Torres GJ, et al. Meta-analyses: key parenting program components for disruptive child behavior. J Am Acad Child Adolesc Psychiatry 2019;58(2):180–90.

41. Epstein RA, Fonnesbeck C, Potter S, et al. Psychosocial interventions for child disruptive behaviors: a meta-analysis. Pediatrics 2015;138(5):947–60.

42. Eyberg SM, Nelson MM, Boggs SR. Evidence-based psychosocial treatments for children and adolescents with disruptive behavior. J Clin Child Adolesc Psychol 2008;37(1):215–37.

43. Farmer EMZ, Compton SN, Burns BJ, et al. Review of the evidence base for treatment of childhood psychopathology: externalizing disorders. J Consult Clin Psychol 2002;70(6):1267 302.

44. Berkout OV, Gross AM. Externalizing behavior challenges in primary care settings. Aggression Violent Behav 2013;18:491–5.

45. Olfson M, Gameroff MJ, Marcus SC, et al. National trends in the treatment of attention deficit hyperactivity disorder. Am J Psychiatry 2003;160(6):1071 7.

46. Danielson ML, Bitsko RH, Ghandour RM, et al. Prevalence of parent-reported ADHD diagnosis and associated treatment among U.S. children and adolescents, 2016. J Clin Child Adolesc Psychol 2018;47(2):199–212.

47. Wolraich ML, Hagan JF, Allan C, et al. Clinical practice guideline for the diagnosis, evaluation, and treatment of attention-deficit/hyperactivity disorder in children and adolescents. Pediatrics 2019;144(4):e20192528.

48. Fabiano GA, Pelham WE, Coles EK, et al. A meta-analysis of behavioral treatments for attention-deficit/hyperactivity disorder. Clin Psychol Rev 2009;29: 129–40.

49. The MTA Cooperative Group. A 14-month randomized clinical trial of treatment strategies for attention-deficit/hyperactivity disorder. Arch Gen Psychiatry 1999; 56:1073–86.

50. Murray DW, Arnold E, Swanson J, et al. A clinical review of outcomes of the multimodal treatment study of children with attention-deficit/hyperactivity disorder (MTA). Curr Psychiatry Rep 2008;10:424–31.

51. Barkley RA. The important role of executive functioning and self-regulation in ADHD. 2012. Available at: http://www.russellbarkley.org/factsheets/ADHD_EF_and_SR.pdf. Accessed July 24, 2020.

52. Barkley RA. Taking chard of ADHD: the complete, authoritative guide for parents. third edition. New York, NY: Guilford Press; 2013.

53. American Academy of Pediatrics (AAP). Caring for children with ADHD: a practical resource toolkit for clinicians. third edition. AAP; 2019.

54. Merikangas KR, He J, Burstein M, et al. Lifetime prevalence of mental disorders in U.S. adolescents: results from the national comorbidity survey replication – adolescent supplement (NCS-A). J Am Acad Child Adolesc Psychiatry 2010; 49(10):980–9.

55. Birmaher B, Khetarpal S, Brent D, et al. The screen for child anxiety related emotional disorders (SCARED): scale construction and psychometric characteristics. J Am Acad Child Adolesc Psychiatry 1997;36(4):545–53.
56. Spitzer RL, Kroenke K, Williams JBW, et al. A brief measure for assessing generalized anxiety disorder. Arch Intern Med 2006;166:1092–7.
57. Barlow DH. Anxiety and its disorders: the nature and treatment of anxiety and panic. New York, NY: Guilford; 2002.
58. Deacon BJ, Abramowitz JS. Cognitive and behavioral treatments for anxiety disorders: a review of meta-analytic findings. J Clin Psychol 2004;60(4):429–41.
59. James AC, James G, Cowdrey FA, et al. Cognitive behavioural therapy for anxiety disorders in children and adolescents. Cochrane Database Syst Rev 2015;2: CD004690.
60. Banneyer KN, Bonin L, Price K, et al. Cognitive behavioral therapy for childhood anxiety disorders: a review of recent advances. Curr Psychiatry Rep 2018;20:65.
61. Kendall PC, Hedtke KA. Cognitive-behavioral therapy for anxious children: therapist manual. third edition. Workbook Publishing; 2006.
62. Kendall PC. Treating anxiety disorders in children: results of a randomized clinical trial. J Consult Clin Psychol 1994;62(1):100–10.
63. Kendall PC, Flannery-Schroeder E, Panichelli-Mindell S, et al. Therapy for youths with anxiety disorders: a second randomized clinical trial. J Consult Clin Psychol 1997;65(3):366–80.
64. Craske MG, Treanor M, Conway CC, et al. Maximizing exposure therapy: an inhibitory learning approach. Behav Res Ther 2014;58:10–23.
65. Weersing VR, Brent DA, Rozenman MS, et al. Brief behavioral therapy for pediatric anxiety and depression in primary care: a randomized clinical trial. JAMA Psychiatry 2017;74(6):571–8.
66. Brent DA, Porta G, Rozenman MS, et al. Brief behavioral therapy for pediatric anxiety and depression in primary care: a follow-up. J Am Acad Child Adolesc Psychiatry 2020;59(7):856–67.
67. Walkup JT, Albano AM, Piacentini J, et al. Cognitive behavioral therapy, sertraline, or a combination in childhood anxiety. N Engl J Med 2008;359(26):2753–66.
68. Pediatric OCD Treatment Study (POTS) Team. Cognitive-behavior therapy, sertraline, and their combination for children and adolescents with obsessive-compulsive disorder: the pediatric OCD treatment study (POTS) randomized controlled trial. JAMA 2004;292(16):1969–76.
69. American Academy of Child and Adolescent Psychiatry. Practice parameter for the assessment and treatment of children and adolescents with anxiety disorders. J Am Acad Child Adolesc Psychiatry 2007;46(2):267–83.
70. Merikangas KR, He JP, Brody D, et al. Prevalence and treatment of mental disorders among U.S. children in the 2001-2004 NHANES. Pediatrics 2010;125(1): 75–81.
71. Kessler RC, Avenolt A, Costello J, et al. Prevalence, persistence, and sociodemographic correlates of DSM-IV disorders in the national comorbidity survey replication adolescent supplement. Arch Gen Psychiatry 2012;69(4):372–80.
72. Kessler RC, Avenevoli S, Ries Merikangas K. Mood disorders in children and adolescents: an epidemiologic perspective. Biol Psychiatry 2001;49(12):1002–14.
73. Zuckerbrot RA, Cheung A, Jensen PS, et al. Guidelines for adolescent depression in primary care (GLAD-PC): Part I. Practice preparation, identification, assessment, and initial management. Pediatrics 2018;141(3):e20174081.
74. Kroenke K, Spitzer RL, Williams JBW. The patient health questionnaire-2: validity of a two-item depression screener. Med Care 2003;41(11):1284–92.

75. Kroenke K, Spitzer RL. The PHQ-9: a new depression diagnostic and severity measure. Psychiatr Ann 2002;32(9):509–15.
76. Faulstich ME, Carey MP, Ruggiero L, et al. Assessment of depression in childhood and adolescence: an evaluation of the Center for Epidemiological Studies Depression Scale for Children (CES-DC). Am J Psychiatry 1986;143:1024–7.
77. Ferster CB. A functional analysis of depression. Am Psychol 1973;28(10):857–70.
78. Lewinsohn PM, Hoberman HM, Teri L, et al. An integrative theory of depression. In: Reiss S, Bootzin RR, editors. Theoretical issues in behavior therapy. New York: Academic Press; 1985. p. 331–59.
79. Martell CR, Addis ME, Jacobson NS. Depression in context: strategies for guided action. New York: W.W. Norton; 2001.
80. Sturmey P. Behavioral activation is an evidence-based treatment for depression. Behav Modif 2009;33(6):818–29.
81. Kanter JW, Manos RC, Bowe WM, et al. What is behavioral activation? A review of the empirical literature. Psychol Rev 2010;30:608–20.
82. Gaynor ST, Harris A. Single-participant assessment of treatment mediators: strategy description and examples from a behavioral activation intervention for depressed adolescents. Behav Modif 2008;32:372–402.
83. McCauley E, Schloredt K, Gudmundsen G, et al. Expanding behavioral activation to depressed adolescents: Lessons learned in treatment development. Cogn Behav Pract 2011;18:371–83.
84. Ritschel LA, Ramirez CL, Jones M, et al. Behavioral activation for depressed teens: a pilot study. Cogn Behav Pract 2011;18:281–99.
85. McCauley E, Gudmundsen G, Schloredt K, et al. The adolescent behavioral activation program: adapting behavioral activation as a treatment for depression in adolescence. J Clin Child Adolesc Psychol 2016;45(3):291–304.
86. Petts RA, Foster CS, Douleh TN, et al. Measuring activation in adolescent depression: preliminary psychometric data on the behavioral activation for depression scale-short form. Behav Anal Res Pract 2016;16(2):65–80.
87. Cheung AH, Zuckerbrot RA, Jensen PS, et al. Guidelines for adolescent depression in primary care (GLAD-PC): Part II. Treatment and ongoing management. Pediatrics 2018;141(3):e20174082.
88. Clarke G, Debar L, Lynch F, et al. A randomized effectiveness trial of brief cognitive-behavioral therapy for depressed adolescents receiving antidepressant medications. J Am Acad Child Adolesc Psychiatry 2005;44(9):888–9.
89. Wright DR, Haaland WL, Ludman E, et al. The costs and cost-effectiveness of collaborative care for adolescents with depression in primary care settings: a randomized clinical trial. JAMA Pediatr 2016;170(11):1048–54.
90. Treatment for Adolescents with Depression Study (TADS) Team. Fluoxetine, cognitive-behavioral therapy, and their combination for adolescents with depression: treatment for adolescents with depression study (TADS) randomized controlled trial. JAMA 2004;292(7):807–20.
91. March JS, Silva S, Petrycki S, et al. The treatment for adolescents with depression study (TADS): long-term effectiveness and safety outcomes. Arch Gen Psychiatry 2007;64(10):1132–43.
92. Kennard BD, Silva SG, Tonev S. Remission and recovery in the treatment for adolescents with depression study (TADS): acute and long-term outcomes. J Am Acad Child Adolesc 2009;48(2):186–95.
93. Substance Abuse and Mental Health Services Administration. Key substance use and mental health indicators in the United States: results from the 2018 national survey on drug Use and health (HHS Publication No. PEP19-5068, NSDUH Series

H-54). Rockville (MD): Center for Behavioral Health Statistics and Quality, Substance Abuse and Mental Health Services Administration; 2019. Available at: https://www.samhsa.gov/data/.

94. Committee on Substance Use and Prevention. Substance use screening, brief intervention, and referral to treatment. Pediatrics 2016;138(1):e20161210.

95. Levy SJL, Williams JF, Committee on Substance Use and Prevention. Substance use screening, brief intervention, and referral to treatment – clinical report. Pediatrics 2016;138(1):e20161211.

96. Levy S, Weiss R, Sherritt L, et al. An electronic screen for triaging adolescent substance use by risk levels. JAMA Pediatr 2014;168(9):822–8.

97. Kelly SM, Gryczynksi J, Mitchell SG, et al. Validity of brief screening instrument for adolescent tobacco, alcohol, and drug use. Pediatrics 2014;133(3):819–26.

98. Miller WR, Rollnick S. Motivational interviewing: preparing people for change. second edition. New York: Guilford Press; 2002.

99. Naar-King S, Suarez M. Motivational interviewing with adolescents and young adults. New York: Guilford Press; 2011.

Ethical and Professional Considerations in Integrated Behavioral Health

Tyler S. Gibb, JD, PhD[a],*, Parker Crutchfield, PhD[a],
Michael J. Redinger, MD, MA[b], John Minser, MFA[a]

KEYWORDS

- Ethics • Professionalism • Integrated behavioral health • Teamwork
- Communication

KEY POINTS

- Integrated behavioral health (IBH) models of care rely on professional and ethical norms from each of the constituent professions, generally with positive results.
- When conflicts arise between the professional and ethical norms of the members of IBH teams, a framework for prioritizing the different interests and obligations is necessary.
- As a rule of thumb, the professional and ethical norms that tend to offer great patient protections ought to be prioritized.
- If possible, discussing potential conflicting norms in a multidisciplinary dialogue will aid in avoiding conflicts.

INTRODUCTION

Despite the clear professional consensus about the overall benefits of integrated behavioral health (IBH) into primary care medicine and endorsement of the model by various agencies,[1–3] little has been written about the related ethical challenges in either the adult or pediatric setting.[4] The few who have written on the topic have identified no shortage of interesting ethical dilemmas, primarily focused on issues such as confidentiality, professional competence, dual relationships, and appropriate boundaries. The literature indicates that those practicing within IBH models are managing ethical conflicts on an ad hoc basis using the collective wisdom and perspectives of those at clinic without the benefit of careful ethical analysis or guidance. Distinctive

[a] Program in Medical Ethics, Humanities & Law, Western Michigan University Homer Stryker M. D. School of Medicine, 1000 Oakland Drive, Kalamazoo, MI 49008-8010, USA; [b] Department of Psychiatry, Program in Medical Ethics, Humanities & Law, Western Michigan University Homer Stryker M.D. School of Medicine, 1000 Oakland Drive, Kalamazoo, MI 49008-8010, USA
* Corresponding author.
E-mail address: tyler.gibb@med.wmich.edu
Twitter: @tsgibb (T.S.G.); @MikeRedingerMD (M.J.R.)

Pediatr Clin N Am 68 (2021) 607–619
https://doi.org/10.1016/j.pcl.2021.02.004
0031-3955/21/© 2021 Elsevier Inc. All rights reserved.

to IBH, conflicts seem arise to when practice habits, clinical guidelines, or policies of 1 member of the multidisciplinary team run afoul of the ethical or professional norms of a team member from a different discipline. Although traditional ethically complex issues exist in IBH, many of the conflicts are interprofessional but also intrateam.[5] This article provides a theoretic and practical framework for IBH practitioners to identify current and potential ethical conflicts in practice, critically reflect on their roles and responsibilities, and offer recommendations on how to address the conflicts unique to the IBH model.

In order to provide ethically sound recommendations, the authors' framework begins by examining the theoretic foundation for the IBH model. It specifically responds to the question: What ethical justification exists for IBH, and what unique benefit does it claim to offer? By providing a robust ethical justification for IBH, this article will then examine some the inherent ethical challenges unique to the IBH model. The source of significant ethical conflict stems from the fact that each member of the IBH team will bring his or her own professional norms, expectations, obligations, and practice standards. For example, a pediatric primary care physician may have a different practice standard for maintaining the confidentiality of sensitive health information than a psychiatrist, psychologist, or social worker from mental health backgrounds. Which set of professional norms should be applied in the pluralistic interdisciplinary IBH model? This article examines a series of issues where professional norms of the various professionals in the IBH model may conflict. With the ultimate goal of providing that which best serves the aim and ethos of IBH, especially applied to the pediatric population, the authors offer recommendations of which professional norms should be adopted by the entire IBH team. Also, this article discusses some of the unique settings where IBH is likely to be implemented and the related ethical challenges.

DISCUSSION
Ethical Justification of Integrated Behavioral Health

Before delving into the competing professional and ethical norms associated with the various health care professions in IBH, one must identify and examine the ethically relevant justifications for IBH itself. If IBH is a superior model of health care, which the authors argue it is, which ethical goals is it more successful in achieving than other models of care? IBH is an integrated system of care that seeks to discharge 2 primary ethical duties: first, improving access to care among the more vulnerable segments of the communities, and, second, increasing the quality of that care.

Accessing high-quality health care is a significant challenge for many families, particularly in communities with fewer resources.[6] The economic and logistical burdens of merely traveling to a health care provider, irrespective of the cost of the care needed, is insurmountable for many families.[7] In situations where the ideal care requires multiple health care providers and specialists, these logistical burdens are compounded.[8] Taking time away from employment, using public transportation, requiring working vehicles with valid registration and licenses, and finding child care are barriers that fall disproportionately on the lower socioeconomic strata of communities. IBH reduces both the number of visits to health care providers and the number of locations that patients and families must visit to receive optimal care. Locating the providers in the same physical location breaks down a significant barrier to accessing health care.

Patients and families will experience little benefit if the health care that is available to them is of marginal quality. Regardless of which normative framework is employed (eg, deontology, consequentialism, teleology, or liberal egalitarianism or communitarianism) providing more access to low-quality health care does not discharge the ethical duty owed patients.[9] IBH aims to not only increase the access, but to also provide a higher quality of care. Communication inefficiencies, administrative redundancies, lack of coordination between providers, and inconsistent follow-up all decrease the quality of health care. IBH, by breaking down barriers to communication between health care providers, reduces the potential for errors in information exchange. Similarly, increasing coordination, fostering interprofessional collaboration, and reducing administrative redundancies also improve the quality of care available.

IBH improves on current models of care by increasing the access to high-quality health care, specifically in communities traditionally marginalized by the health care system.

Examining the Various Ethical Norms in Integrated Behavioral Health

Ethical issues arise in any clinical setting, but when integrating behavioral health into the ordinary operations of outpatient care, ethical concerns emerge in unique ways, and may require a different approach. Not only are the challenges unique, but there is little clarity on how the ethical challenges may be appropriately addressed, and how one might prioritize competing professional norms. For example, concerns about when and how a health care provider must break the confidentiality between provider and patient are approached differently by the professional norms of social workers and the professional norms of psychiatrists.[4] In these types of situations where professional norms do not align or directly conflict, which profession's norms ought to take precedence? There is little guidance on this question. Some professional norms are very protective of the patient's rights (eg, mental health providers). Other professional norms seem to prioritize community benefit over an individual patient's interests (eg, community health nursing). Within a multidisciplinary IBH team, there are situations where 1 professional norm seems most appropriate, but other times an ethical norm from another profession feels most appropriate. The goals and efficacy of IBH are evident, but the uncertainty of prioritizing and harmonizing professional norms must be addressed.

In the following sections, the authors propose a framework for prioritizing various, and sometimes competing, professional norms operating in IBH. The proposed framework characterizes professional norms in 3 ways, focusing on their prioritization of patients' rights: very protective of patient rights, moderately protective of patient rights, and those norms in which other rights and interests are treated equally as other priorities (eg, public safety). These categorizations will be explained through careful examination of a series of topics that cause ethical consternation for health care providers in the IBH model. Any given health care profession (eg, primary care physicians or social workers) may have some norms fall into each of these 3categories. By looking carefully at confidentiality and informed consent, boundary and dual relationship issues, opportunities to engage in research activities, and bias and discrimination concerns, the authors will explore the 3 levels of protection available in the relevant professional norms, then offer a recommendation regarding which level of protection best accomplishes the overall goals of IBH. These recommendations are compiled in a table that follows the discussion (**Table 1**).

Confidentiality

Consider the ethical requirement that providers maintain the confidentiality of patients.[10–12] Confidentiality is the bedrock of the trust required for a functional therapeutic alliance between health care provider and patient. Trust is especially important for

Table 1
Recommendations for conflicting integrated behavioral health professional norms

Confidentiality	• Obtain consent from new patients for sharing information among the care team • Restrict disclosure of health information with those outside the care team
Informed Consent/Assent	• To the extent that it is possible, seek informed consent from parents and patients • Be prepared to presume consent in emergencies or when the benefits strongly outweigh the risks
Boundary and Dual Relationship Issues	• Clinicians should expect to work and interact with members of patient families, both in clinical and community settings • Major conflicts of interest (ie, sexual relationships with patient family members) should be avoided
Opportunities for Research Participation	• Research is necessary for investigation of best practices and efficacy • Implement heightened protection for patients because of increased presence of vulnerable populations
Professional Competency	• In all IBH contexts, incentives to overreach professional competence exist; all members of the team should be aware of their roles and limitations, and practice guidelines that limit care to those with appropriate professional competence should be enforced
Implicit Bias	• In general, the negative effects of implicit bias are reduced by IBH; nevertheless, explicit implementation of anti-bias measures is warranted

Unique Practice Setting Issues	• Military
	  ○ Increased awareness of limitations of professional competence
	• Rural settings
	  ○ Increased awareness of increased likelihood of multiple role conflicts and confidentiality breaches
	  ○ Implement processes to ensure professional competency from practice members with flexible roles
	• Education
	  ○ Increased awareness of multiple role conflicts
	  ○ Interpersonal conflicts may be exacerbated by informal consultation, perceptions of professional competency, and fluidity of assessor-learner relationships
	• Patients at end of life
	  ○ Integrated care of multiple family members may lead to conflicts between dying patients and family members who are also patients
	  ○ Attention to documentation and language used in patient interactions can help reduce unintentional breaches of confidentiality
	• Patients with chronic pain
	  ○ Heightened confidentiality procedures may be necessary in order to combat treatment stigma
	  ○ Awareness of difficulties in obtaining informed consent among patients suffering from chronic pain

providers offering behavioral and mental health care to adolescents. Breaking confidentiality can undermine this trust, but there are situations where other goods can only be achieved by violating the confidences shared between health care provider and patient[13,14] (eg, sharing sensitive information with other professionals to facilitate better care, or to ensure access to important resources or sources of support). Thus, the ethical obligation to maintain confidentiality can be overridden by other obligations, increasing the likelihood of successful treatment. Under what circumstances, to whom, and what information may be shared are important questions for all health care providers to answer.

IBH providers from different professional backgrounds may answer these questions in different ways. The varied professional norms prioritize the patient's right to confidentiality in different ways and recommend different best practices, creating different tiers of protection. In the most protective tier, patient confidentiality is vigorously protected. Except in cases when a health care provider has a legal duty to protect others, such as when he or she has a duty to warn others of a potential threat, those providing mental health care disclose patient information to no one, not even other providers, without explicit consent from the patient.[15] In the least protective tier, typical of professionals in public health, confidentiality is guarded, but certain disclosures about a patient's health are not only permissible, but obligatory, such as when a patient has a sexually transmitted infection or one or more of various qualifying infectious diseases. The health and safety of the public is a serious consideration.

The middle tier of protection maintains strict confidentiality between patient and the health care team—disclosure of information to those outside of the team requires explicit consent from the patient. However, it presumes consent for disclosure of information within the team itself. For example, primary care providers presume consent for the sharing of information with nurses, some office staff, other primary care doctors, specialists, and other medical professionals. This balances confidentiality with providing quality care to the patient. Or, to put it another way, this tier of protection best facilitates quality care in that setting because it allows the free flow of information.

Given the goal of integrating behavioral health into primary care is to increase the quality of care a patient receives, the tier of protection that best facilitates this aim is the middle tier. In settings with IBH, the interprofessional sharing of information allows each professional to use and share that information to provide better care within the team. However, this tier of protection also restricts the disclosure of information to those outside the team, maintaining confidentiality and the trust that it grounds. This approach may feel too lax for psychiatrists, for example, or too restrictive, for community-based epidemiologists. But a balance of patient rights and free flow of information is the goal.

For example, suppose a 15-year-old boy speaks with a family medicine physician in a clinic with an IBH provider. The boy says things indicating depression, but that he does not want his parents to know about what he is feeling. In such a setting, the best care is likely to involve the behavioral health professional, and presumed consent for disclosure most efficiently facilitates that person's involvement (although presumed consent does not obviate a discussion with the boy about behavioral health services or his consent for treatment). The interprofessional sharing of information, however, does not require explicit disclosure to his parents.

Informed consent
The tiers of protection also help guide ethical practices in honoring the patient's autonomy. The honoring of patient autonomy is most efficiently achieved by acquiring informed consent for treatment, which is a process of education and shared decision

making between the provider and the patient, or, in the case of minors, the provider, the patient, and the parent.[16–18] The first tier of professional norms offers the highest degree of protection of the patient's autonomy and closely makes virtually no leeway to presume consent to treatment. With the exception of rare and specific cases (eg, involuntary commitment or an emergency), this tier of protection recommends that nothing be done to or for a patient without the actual and informed consent of the patient or his or her legally authorized decision maker.[19,20]

The second tier of protection allows for consent for some treatments to be presumed or implied. These cases include implicit consent when changing prescriptions while hospitalized, or, in pediatric patients, when the benefits so strongly outweigh the risks of a discrete, life-saving intervention. In virtually all other cases, however, informed consent from the parent or patient must be acquired. The third tier of professional norms is the least restrictive, allowing for greater exceptions to informed consent. These occur most frequently in the public health setting, such as with the compulsory administration of vaccinations or in cases of isolation techniques like quarantine.[21–23]

Acquiring informed consent is a good thing.[24] There is almost no situation in which achieving informed consent is worse than not having achieved it.[25,26] To the extent possible, it should be sought in all cases, and integrating behavioral health into the care of a patient does not change this obligation. Unless a patient satisfies one of the previously mentioned conditions (needs emergency care, is hospitalized, or lacks the capacity to make his or her own decisions for treatment and the benefits strongly outweigh the risks), there is no reason for a physician or IBH professional to presume or infer consent to be treated. That is, integrating behavioral health into primary care practices does not create new situations in which presuming or inferring consent is justifiable.[27,28] Further, because IBH often represents a patient's first encounter with behavioral health professionals, there is no history of a patient's having a trusting relationship with such professionals. A thorough informed consent process can encourage trust, ensure the development of a healthy, robust therapeutic alliance, and improve the overall quality of care. Practicing in accordance with the first tier of protection ensures that this takes place.

Boundary and dual relationships

Mental health professionals who come to the practice of IBH will likely bring with them a heightened sensitivity regarding boundary and dual relationship issues.[29,30] Mental health has a long history of recognizing that the actions of the mental health professional may have increased influence over patients, in part because of the more intimate nature of the relationship that forms between patients and their therapists or psychiatrists. Normal unconscious feelings directed toward the mental health professional, referred to as transference, often reflect previous experiences with persons from the patient's past.[31,32] These unintentional emotions place patients at higher risk of exploitation by those working with them on sensitive issues. Additionally, unconscious, unintentional feelings also reflexively arise from the therapist toward the patient and are referred to as countertransference. They, too, increase the risk of a boundary violation, or when the mental health professional either intentionally or unintentionally exploits a patient for personal gain. As a result, mental health professionals are apt to monitor their encounters with patients with increased scrutiny. The ethics codes for both psychiatrists and psychologists extensively address this issue and encourage these professionals to decrease the risk of boundary violations by limiting their involvement, or dual relationships, in the lives of their patients outside of the clinical milieu. Importantly for the pediatric population, they also encourage the same with other third parties associated with child and adolescent patients. For example, they may be more inclined to bank or shop elsewhere than where their adolescent patient's parent works. Contrast this with a primary care pediatrician who may see nothing amiss with conducting routine day-to-day activities they would be doing otherwise that bring them into contact with the parents of their patients.

In the question of which set of professional standards, mental health or primary care, better advance the goals of IBH, it may be that adhering to increased caution in boundary and dual relationship issues as in mental health may not be feasible, if not impossible. Whereas a mental health professional usually declines to treat members of the same family, this likely would inhibit the ability of an IBH clinic to achieve its aims of increasing access to behavioral health care. Likewise, in rural areas, it may place an unreasonable burden on IBH clinicians to ask all of them to grocery shop in the next town over because a patient's father works as the butcher. Certainly, this does not mean that all IBH clinicians should see this advice as license to pursue relationships that they would normally shy away from, such as sexual relationships with family members of a current patient. However, when developing policies or procedures pertaining to interactions between IBH practitioners, patients, and their family members, the clinic may be ethically justified in erring on the side of allowing actions aimed at increasing health care access and quality.

Opportunities for research

Continuous research is critical to the provision of high-quality health care and the development of new, effective treatments. This is particularly relevant in the IBH setting where efficacy and best practices continue to be verified and defined.[33] There is no 1 type of research that can advance these goals in isolation and scholars from a vast array of disciplines, with a variety methodologies and tools, are necessary. However, these diverse academic backgrounds bring along a diverse set of practices and ethical norms, which may create conflict or concern. Regardless of the setting or the type of research being performed, clinical trials of new medications, ethnographic studies of groups of people or places, or statistical evaluations of disease burden, these activities should fall under the auspices of human subjects research protection programs. HRPP, most commonly encountered through the IRB application process, had the mandate to regulate research on human subjects with the ultimate goal of protecting participants. The amount of scrutiny that the HRPP applies, and the amount of regulation imposed, depends on the type of research (degree of risk to participants), but also the characteristics of the research participants involved (eg, minors or prisoners). Social science researchers, for example, may be accustomed to much laxer HRPP regulation than researchers doing clinical drug trials. However, the important ethical question is how strictly should HRPP regulate research on this population and in these practice areas?

Patient and families who seek treatment in an IBH clinic will be the subjects of much research in the future, which the authors unequivocally support. Best practices need to be evaluated and defined, and efficacy needs to be demonstrated. Although not explicitly listed as one of the vulnerable populations requiring heightened protections in the federal regulations, the authors argue that research on IBH patient and in IBH settings should be strictly regulated.[34] Patients seeking treatment at IBH clinics are more likely to be facing a combination of economic and social barriers to treatment; there tends to be a history of lack of access and marginalization, and the type of treatment being provided (ie, mental health treatment), leaves them more vulnerable to research misconduct.[35] It is unlikely that the federal regulations will be amended to include this specific population in the formal rules, but local HRPP and IRB can provide heightened protections for this setting.

Implicit bias

Health care professionals across scopes of practice are as likely as the wider population to display implicit bias based on characteristics such as race, gender, and socioeconomic status.[36] Perceived dangerousness of mental health patients has also been identified as an important bias and is a major component of mental health service use stigma.[37] Because of the characteristics of the patient population at clinical sites currently implementing IBH and the integration of care into a single medical home, unexamined biases may have significant implications for equity and quality of care.

Implicit bias has been implicated in multiple examples of care disparity, including dismissal of pain scale reporting in Black patients and major differences in prescription of psychiatric medications among racial groups.[38] Positively, it has been suggested that the dangerousness bias associated with mental health service patients may be reduced by the integration of mental health care with other medical care.[39] Evidence suggests that patients who might otherwise slip through the cracks are more likely to receive mental health care at a practice that has implemented IBH.[40] Explicit implementation of anti-bias measures is strongly recommended.

Unique Settings for Integrated Behavioral Health

A recent periodic reviewed the applicability of several codes of ethics to particular IBH settings, with authors in some case clarifying the applicability of existing codes to common situations in IBH, and in others recommending adjustments to codes.[41] These articles paid particular attention to how the guidelines of the American Psychological Association interacted with other professional codes. The recommendations presented, however, were applicable to the entire IBH clinic.

Military

Dobmeyer raises 2 concerns about IBH in military settings: first, that military culture privileges just-in-time training and flexibility, which may encourage providers to take on tasks that go beyond the limits of their professional competence; and second, that small base settings may contribute to multiple role conflicts. As Gould points out, resource limitations may mean making a decision that puts the beneficence/nonmaleficence principle in conflict with the justice principle.[42] In addition, Owen and Wanzer warn that military settings are at particular risk for compassion fatigue among health care team members, which may contribute to violations of the justice principle if equality of care is not maintained because of provider fatigue.[43]

In military settings, professionals (such as chaplains and social workers) are frequently called upon to provide mental health support that may go beyond the bounds of their training.[41,44] To address this concern, the authors recommend practice-wide awareness of scopes of practice, accompanied by written guidelines and checklists where established procedures exist. In emerging fields of practice where best practices have not been robustly developed, the authors concur with Dobmeyer's recommendation that all members of the team recognize limitations and uncertainties and to take appropriate steps to ensure the competence of their work. As in many other contexts, the possibility of multiple role conflict is real, and although medium-tier protections can help to minimize the possibility of entering inappropriate personal or financial relationships with current patients, in high-uncertainty situations, the boundaries between personal friends or colleagues and potential patients can shift rapidly.

Rural settings

Mullin and Stenger raise 3 ethical concerns common to rural practice: multiple roles conflicts, confidentiality, and competence,[45] some of which have already been explicitly addressed. Because of the close-knit character of rural communities, irreducible conflicts between the needs of patients can easily arise in the normal course of practice.[8] The potential harm of multiple relationships is compounded by the nature of information flow in rural communities, where therapeutic details may become known through community activity, and where attempts to secure consent to discuss therapy with others may itself represent a breach of confidentiality, as in cases where 2 closely related patients share the same providers. Finally, providers may not have the resources available to refer patients to specialists and may be called upon to perform procedures or therapies outside their scope of competence. Mullin and Stenger's recommendation relating to professional competence – that providers do not need to attempt to do it alone and may benefit from reaching out to specialists, colleagues, and professional societies for training – is a fine reminder for providers worried about disclosing a potential ethical concern. Also, utilizing technological advancements may prove beneficial.[7,46] Managing multiple relationships and confidentiality in rural settings requires restricting information whenever possible to those within the care team. In situations where the needs of 2 or more patients are irreconcilable, steps must be taken to resolve the conflict as justly as possible. This may take the form of referrals to colleagues or restrictions to the provider's nonclinical community roles.

Health care education

Health care education in an IBH setting magnifies the opportunity for multiple role conflicts among colleagues and coworkers.[47] Close integration and its attendant free flow of information, coupled with interpersonal feeling on topics of professional competence, scopes of practice, and adversarial or advisory supervisor-trainee relationships, all contribute to potential conflicts of interest regarding student evaluation.[48] Informal consultation, too, poses a particularly challenging potential multiple roles conflict; information acquired from informal settings may impact the formal aspects of collegial or instructor-student relationships, while semiformal care may negatively impact valued informal relationships. The recommendations outlined by Reitz and colleagues, suggest that because the faculty role in medical education is composed of both advisory functions (ie, mentorship) and adversarial functions (ie, evaluation and gatekeeping), it is more practical and effective for faculty to steer a middle course with regard to their personal, clinical, and service/fiscal relationships than it is to attempt to limit which of the faculty functions they engage in with particular students and colleagues. They suggest aiming for friendly, collegial personal relationships, frank informal health advice that does not enter a doctor-patient relationship, and general personal assistance that avoids contractual fiscal partnership. This aligns with the authors' recommendation for middle-tier protections that acknowledge the inevitability of multiple roles while avoiding those conflicts of interest that are likely to compromise objectivity and good clinical and evaluative judgment.

End of life

For providers who are caring for a dying patient alongside members of that patient's family, ethical conflicts related to who is being treated may arise.[49] Mental health support given to members of a dying patient's family may involve discussion – or withheld discussion – of details of the patient's condition depending on patient and familial preferences. The decision to end treatment may also be fraught, especially for members of historically oppressed groups, which may erode trust in the practice for the entire surviving family.[49] The conflict between patient autonomy and the need to provide equitable, high-quality care to all patients, including family members of patients, may create situations in which clinicians' multiple roles demand differing goals. The authors endorse Gould's recommendation of clear documentation, including Rosenberg and Spiece's call for "patient reports" language, in order to best provide care while reducing opportunities for violations of confidentiality. When feasible, referrals to other appropriate partners can help minimize the potential of major conflicts.

Patients with chronic pain

Access to appropriate pain management is a growing issue across the continuum of care.[50] Robinson and Rickard describe ways in which patients with chronic pain may be more vulnerable than others with regard to obtaining informed consent and maintaining beneficence/nonmaleficence.[51–53] Implicit bias may also play a role in determining which patients receive pain medication and which do not. Their recommendation that written materials describing the benefits and drawbacks of narcotic pain medication be provided is appropriate, although patient health literacy will play a major role in the effectiveness of such materials. Strict confidentiality should be maintained, since stigma associated with narcotic pain management and addictive behavior may undermine therapeutic relationships.

SUMMARY

This article intended to

> Provide an ethical rationale for the IBH model grounded in increasing patient access to care and improving quality of care
> Explore an ethical framework in managing ethical dilemmas that occur in IBH by analyzing the protections and restrictions provided to patients by the different ethical norms IBH practitioners may apply from other professions
> Assist in determining which set of norms may be best in meeting the goals of IBH in a pediatric setting
> Propose a set of ethical best practices adaptable by IBH practices

Further research is necessary to identify if this model is successful in assisting IBH practices in resolving the inevitable ethical conflicts that ought to occur as the IBH model continues to grow in influence.

CLINICS CARE POINTS

- New patients should be informed that care information is shared among the health team, and a global consent for information sharing should be obtained.
- EMR barriers designed to limit shared information should be removed, except where required by law.
- Be aware of each state's laws on parental consent and assent.

DISCLOSURE

No financial or relationship conflicts of interest relevant to this publication.

REFERENCES

1. Asarnow JR, Rozenman M, Wiblin J, et al. Integrated medical-behavioral care compared with usual primary care for child and adolescent behavioral health. JAMA Pediatr 2015;169(10):929–37.
2. Balasubramanian BA, Cohen DJ, Jetelina KK, et al. Outcomes of integrated behavioral health with primary care. J Am Board Fam Med 2017;30(2):130–9.
3. Kolko DJ, Perrin E. The Integration of Behavioral Health Interventions in Children's Health Care: Services, Science, and Suggestions. J Clin Child Adolesc Psychol 2014;43(2):216–28.
4. Hudgins C, Rose S, Fifield PY, et al. Navigating the legal and ethical foundations of informed consent and confidentiality in integrated primary care. Fam Syst Health 2013;31(1):9–19.
5. Gamero N, GonzálezRomá V, Peiró JM. The influence of intra-team conflict on work teams' affective climate: a longitudinal study. J Occup Organizational Psychol 2008;81(1):47–69.
6. Institute of Medicine. Challenges and successes in reducing health disparities: workshop summary. Washington, DC: National Academies Press (US); 2008.
7. Grazier KL, Smiley ML, Bondalapati KS. Overcoming Barriers to Integrating Behavioral Health and Primary Care Services. J Prim Care Community Health 2016;7(4):242–8.
8. Eberhardt MS, Pamuk ER. The Importance of Place of Residence: Examining Health in Rural and Nonrural Areas. Am J Public Health 2011;94(10):1682–6.
9. Sugarman J, Sulmasy DP1. Methods in medical ethics. Washington, DC: Georgetown University Press; 2001.
10. Duncan RE, Vandeleur M, Derks A, et al. Confidentiality with adolescents in the medical setting: what do parents think? J Adolesc Health 2011;49(4):428–30.
11. Klein CA. Cloudy confidentiality: clinical and legal implications of cloud computing in health care. J Am Acad Psychiatry Law 2011;39(4):571–8.
12. Purtilo RB, Doherty RF. Why honor confidentiality?. In: Ethical dimensions in the health professions. Boston: Elsevier; 2005. p. 202–21. Available at: https://www.elsevier.com/books/ethical-dimensions-in-the-health-professions/purtilo/978-1-4557-3684-3.
13. Barnard D. Vulnerability and Trustworthiness. Cambridge Q Healthc Ethics 2016; 25(02):288–300.
14. Busch JS, Hantusch N. I don't trust you, but why don't you trust me? Dispute Resolution J 2000;55(3):56–65.
15. Rothstein MA. Tarasoff Duties after Newtown. J Law Med Ethics 2014;42(1): 104–9.
16. Cocanour CS. Informed consent-It's more than a signature on a piece of paper. Am J Surg 2017;214(6):993–7.
17. Meisel A, Kuczewski MG. Legal and ethical myths about informed consent. Arch Intern Med 1996;156(22):2521–6.
18. Waltz JR, Scheuneman TW. Informed consent to therapy. Nw UL Rev 1969;64(5): 628–50.
19. Chow GV. CURVES: a mnemonic for determining medical decision-making capacity and providing emergency treatment in the acute setting. Chest 2010; 137(2):421–7.
20. Pope TM. Legal fundamentals of surrogate decision making. Chest 2012;141(4): 1074–81.

21. Bostick NA, Levine MA, Sade RM. Ethical obligations of physicians participating in public health quarantine and isolation measures. Public Health Rep 2008; 123(1):3–8.
22. Giubilini A, Douglas T, Maslen H, et al. Quarantine, isolation and the duty of easy rescue in public. Dev World Bioeth 2017;18(2):182–9.
23. Pope TM, Bughman HM. Legal briefing: coerced treatment and involuntary confinement for contagious disease. J Clin Ethics 2015;26(1):73–83.
24. Eyal N. Informed Consent (Stanford Encyclopedia of Philosophy) [Internet]. Stanford Encyclopedia of Philosophy. 2015. pp. 1–21. Available at: https://plato.stanford.edu/cgi-bin/encyclopedia/archinfo.cgi?entry=informed-consent.   Accessed October 16, 2015.
25. American Academy of Pediatrics Committee on Bioethics. Informed consent in decision-making in pediatric practice. Pediatrics 2016;138(2). e20161484–4.
26. Levy N. Forced to be free? Increasing patient autonomy by constraining it. J Med Ethics 2014;40:293–300.
27. Cole CA. Implied consent and nursing practice: ethical or convenient? Nurs Ethics 2012;19(4):550–7.
28. McCullough LB, McGuire AL, Whitney SN. Consent: informed, simple, implied and presumed. Am J Bioeth 2007;7(12):49–50 [discussion: W3–4].
29. Glover JJ. Rural bioethical issues of the elderly: how do they differ from urban ones? J Rural Health 2001;17(4):332–5.
30. Nadelson C, Notman MT. Boundaries in the doctor-patient relationship. Theor Med Bioeth 2002;23(3):191–201.
31. Jones AC. Transference, counter-transference and repetition: some implications for nursing practice. J Clin Nurs 2005;14(10):1177–84.
32. Simon RI. Treatment boundary violations: clinical, ethical, and legal considerations. Bull Am Acad Psychiatry Law 1992;20(3):269–88.
33. Campbell-Page RM, Shaw-Ridley M. Managing ethical dilemmas in community-based participatory research with vulnerable populations. Health Promot Pract 2013;14(4):485–90.
34. Waisel DB. Vulnerable populations in healthcare. Curr Opin Anaesthesiol 2013; 26(2):186–92.
35. DuBois JM, Anderson EE, Carroll K, et al. Environmental factors contributing to wrongdoing in medicine: a criterion-based review of studies and cases. Ethics & Behav 2012;22(3):163–88.
36. FitzGerald C, Hurst S. Implicit bias in healthcare professionals: a systematic review. BMC Med Ethics 2017;18(1):19.
37. Watson AC, Corrigan PW, Angell B, et al. What Motivates Public Support for Legally Mandated Mental Health Treatment? Social Work Res 2005;29(2):87–94.
38. Hoffman KM, Trawalter S, Axt JR, et al. Racial bias in pain assessment and treatment recommendations, and false beliefs about biological differences between blacks and whites. Proc Natl Acad Sci U S A Natl Acad Sci 2016;113(16): 4296–301.
39. Sowislo JF, Gonet-Wirz F, Borgwardt S, et al. Perceived dangerousness as related to psychiatric symptoms and psychiatric service use – a vignette based representative population. Surv Scientific Rep 2017;7(1):45716.
40. Bridges AJ, Gregus SJ, Rodriguez JH, et al. Diagnoses, intervention strategies, and rates of functional improvement in integrated behavioral health care patients. J Consult Clin Psychol 2015;83(3):590–601.
41. Dobmeyer AC. Primary care behavioral health: ethical issues in military settings. Fam Syst Health 2013;31(1):60–8.

42. Gould DA. Primary care provider reflections on context-specific quandaries from special issue on ethical quandaries when delivering integrated primary care. Fam Syst Health 2013;31(1):84–5.
43. Owen RP, Wanzer L. Compassion fatigue in military healthcare teams. Arch Psychiatr Nurs 2014;28(1):2–9.
44. Kopacz MS, Nieuwsma JA, Jackson GL, et al. Chaplains' engagement with suicidality among their service users: findings from the VA/DoD Integrated Mental Health Strategy. Suicide Life-Threatening Behav 2016;46(2):206–12.
45. Mullin D, Stenger J. Ethical matters in rural integrated primary care settings. Fam Syst Health 2013;31(1):69–74.
46. Suttle A. Using Technology to improve rural health care. Harvard Business Review; 2017. p. 1–5.
47. Hoeft TJ, Fortney JC, Patel V, et al. Task-sharing approaches to improve mental health care in rural and other low-resource settings: a systematic review. J Rural Health 2018;34(1):48–62.
48. Reitz R, Simmons PD, Runyan C, et al. Multiple role relationships in healthcare education. Fam Syst Health 2013;31(1):96–107.
49. Rosenberg T, Speice J. Integrating care when the end is near: ethical dilemmas in end-of-life care. Fam Syst Health 2013;31(1):75–83.
50. Shipton EA, Shipton EE, Shipton AJ. A Review of the Opioid Epidemic: What Do We Do About It? Pain Ther 2018;7(1):23–36.
51. DeMonte CM, DeMonte WD, Thorn BE. Future implications of eHealth interventions for chronic pain management in underserved populations. Pain Manag 2015;5(3):207–14.
52. Robinson PJ, Rickard JA. Ethical quandaries in caring for primary-care patients with chronic pain. Fam Syst Health 2013;31(1):52–9.
53. Harrison JM, Lagisetty P, Sites BD, et al. Trends in prescription pain medication use by race/ethnicity among US adults with noncancer pain, 2000-2015. Am J Public Health 2018;108(6):788–90.

Pediatric Residency Training for Integration of Behavior Health: Indian Perspective

Swati Y. Bhave, MD, DCH, FCPS, FIAP, FAAP (HON)[a,b,*],
Harish K. Pemde, MD, FIAP[c], Rajesh Mehta, MD[d]

KEYWORDS

- Behavior • Children • Adolescents • Medical education • Residency program

KEY POINTS

- Behavior problems in children and adolescents in India.
- Behavior health in residency programs in pediatrics in India and developed countries.
- Impact of culture on behavioral health of children and adolescents in India.
- Integration of behavioral health of children and adolescents in curriculum in pediatrics residency programs in India.

INTRODUCTION

Mental health problems, including behavioral and psychiatric disorders, are common in children and adolescents. Few studies have reported prevalence of variety of these disorders from India. We could not find a robust study representative of India on behavior or mental health disorders; however, several small studies have reported behavioral and mental health disorders in Indian children.

A recent study on children living in institutional homes reported 1 or more behavioral and emotional problems in 16.78% of the residents, including conduct problems (34.90%), peer problems (15.80%), emotional problems (14.70%), hyperactivity

Dr R. Mehta is a staff member of the World Health Organization. The author alone is responsible for the views expressed in this publication and they do not necessarily represent the decisions or policies of the World Health Organization.
[a] AACCI, Association of Adolescent and Child Care in India, Mumbai, India; [b] Dr D.Y. Patil Medical College, Pimpri, India and Dr.D.Y. Patil Vidyapeeth, Pune, India; [c] Department of Pediatrics, WHO Collaborating Center for Training and Research in Adolescent Health, Lady Hardinge Medical College, Kalawati Saran Children's Hospital, 1, Nav Vikas Apartment Sector 15 Rohini, Delhi 110089 India; [d] Neonatal, Child and Adolescent Health, WHO South East Asia, SP-15 Pitam Pura, Delhi 110034, India
* Corresponding author. AACCI, 302, "Charleville", "A" Road, Churchgate, Mumbai 400 020, Maharashtra, India.
E-mail address: sybhave@gmail.com

(8.60%), and low prosocial behavior (3.40%).[1] A study on alcohol use among adolescents in Kerala (a state of Southern India) found prevalence of lifetime alcohol use in 15% of adolescents (23.2% among boys and 6.5% among girls; 1 in 4 alcohol users reported hazardous alcohol use; and mean age at onset of alcohol use in adolescents was 13.6 years).[2] One study in the eastern part of India found the overall rate of smoking as 29.6% among adolescents. Among smokers, most (75%) started smoking by 15 years.[3] A recent study found problematic mobile phone use in 6.3% children and adolescents and 16% among adolescents.[4] A systematic review on prevalence of child and adolescent psychiatric disorders in India in 2014 found that overall 6.46% children and adolescents in the community had 1 or other psychiatric disorders, whereas the same was found in 23.33% of school-going children and adolescents.[5] A 2014 review on young people (10–24 years old) in India found health impacting behaviors and conditions in 10% to 30% of young people.[6] These included tobacco use, harmful alcohol use, other substance use, high-risk sexual behaviors, stress, common mental disorders, and injuries (road traffic injuries, suicides, violence of different types). Disorders like pica, temper tantrums, breath-holding space, attention deficit hyperactivity disorder, tobacco use, and substance abuse are common in children and adolescents. Pediatric residents are going to be challenged with such issues and hence they should be trained to become capable of identifying and managing these mental health (behavioral) conditions in their future careers.

INDIA SCENARIO: PEDIATRIC TRAINING IN BACHELOR OF MEDICINE AND BACHELOR OF SURGERY AND POSTGRADUATE PROGRAMS AND INTEGRATION OF BEHAVIORAL HEALTH

Pediatrics was earlier included under the subject of Internal Medicine in India in the undergraduate and postgraduate (PG) curricula. It was introduced as an independent subject in MBBS (undergraduate program in medicine: Bachelor of Medicine and Bachelor of Surgery) only in the early 1990s.The beginning of PG programs in India varied depending on the institutions, and it began in the late 1950s and early 1960s. Both in undergraduate and PG programs, the pediatric curriculum included a significant component of prevention and health promotion, including behavioral determinants of health in terms of nutrition, and personal and environmental hygiene. In addition, growth and development of children is an essential part of the pediatric curriculum and includes behavioral pediatrics as well. In 1999, the Indian Academy of Pediatrics (IAP) made a policy[7] that pediatricians should provide care for children 0 to 18 years of age. The year 2000 was declared as IAP year of Adolescent Health[8] and IAP also started a subspecialty group on adolescent pediatrics. Since then, IAP has been advocating with the government to include adolescent health in the curriculum of MBBS and postgraduate programs. Concerted efforts of adolescent health advocates led to inclusion of "provision of capacity building of health care providers in adolescent health during pre-service training" in strategy handbook of Rashtriya Kishor Swasthya Karyakram, the national program on adolescent health in India in 2014.[9] Recently, in 2019, adolescent health has finally been included in the pediatric curriculum of MBBS across all medical colleges of India.[10] This has paved the way for including behavioral issues of adolescents also. The new curriculum for PG courses (MD in pediatrics) is being implemented by the universities. The PG curriculum has traditionally been very flexible and focused on the problems and diseases of the local population. Somehow, the required focus on adolescent health has been missing in PG training programs and the IAP Adolescent Chapter, now called AHA – Adolescent Health Academy, is making efforts to get this included.

Several health problems in the adolescent health group are directly or indirectly related to unhealthy lifestyle or risk-taking behaviors. for example, obesity, sexually transmitted infections, human immunodeficiency virus, unwanted teen pregnancies, traffic accidents, and injuries. Hence, the integrated behavioral approach, both in undergraduate and PG and residency training programs in pediatrics, will create physicians who are better equipped to handle preventive counseling and anticipatory guidance, which are key factors to address these issues in children and adolescents.

In summary, the theoretic aspects of health prevention and promotion, as well as behavioral health, are reasonably covered in the pediatrics curriculum at undergraduate and PG levels. However, the emphasis on these issues in pediatrics residency programs is inadequate in practical terms. In the pediatric residency training programs, the opportunities to work away from the hospitals and in close cooperation with families and the local community are not adequate. Pediatric residents do not get to practice integrated behavioral health (IBH) principles to improve their competencies in this important aspect of child and adolescent health.

THE SCENARIO IN DEVELOPED COUNTRIES

There is increasing incidence of mental health issues among children and adolescents across the world and adolescents young adults. A Report of the Surgeon General of the United States[11] documents the high prevalence of mental health needs of America's youth. Although almost 1 in 5 children in the United States suffers from a diagnosable mental disorder, only 20% to 25% of affected children receive treatment. This is a troubling statistic, considering that treatment of many mental disorders has been deemed highly effective. The Surgeon General's report highlights the challenges of gaining access to mental health services in a complex and often fragmented system of health care. Without intervention, child and adolescent psychiatric disorders frequently continue into adulthood. For example, research shows that when children with coexisting depression and conduct disorders become adults, they tend to use more health care services and have higher health care costs than other adults. If the system does not appropriately screen and treat them early, these childhood disorders may persist and lead to a downward spiral of school failure, poor employment opportunities, and poverty in adulthood. No other illnesses damage so many children so seriously.[12] Most of these patients are first seen by primary care pediatricians[13–16] It is very important for pediatricians to be trained in mental health issues and work in collaboration with mental health professionals for holistic management of these patients. This is best achieved by an IBH approach during the pediatric residency itself.[17,18] It is equally important that such a concept is also introduced in the psychiatric residency to train them in child and adolescent developmental aspects. Pediatric education in the care for children with behavior and mental health problems includes anticipatory guidance, problem identification, primary care counseling, referral, and collaborative care with a behavioral health professional.[19,20] Developing lasting collaborative relationships with mental health colleagues, making effective referrals, and planning and executing a shared treatment plan across disciplines all require training, skill, and experience.[21]

The American Academy of Pediatrics (AAP) has been periodically issuing statements regarding this aspect.[22–24] In March of 2009, the American Academy of Child and Adolescent Psychiatry and the AAP issued a joint position paper highlighting the importance of addressing the mental health needs of children and adolescents in primary care settings and made recommendations for overcoming financial and administrative barriers to mental health care delivery in primary care. The AAP released its own policy statement in the summer of 2009 discussing the need for advances in residency training, continuing education, and clinician commitment for the provision of mental health care within pediatric primary care.[25]

Garfunkel and colleagues in 2001[26] did a study to compare former pediatric residents' perceptions of their training in behavioral health care and collaboration from 2 separate continuity clinic sites within 1 training program that used either conventional or integrated models of behavioral health care. The results showed total of 174 alumni (71%) returned completed questionnaires. Overall, there were significant differences between graduates in the 2 groups. Residents who trained and practiced alongside behavioral health fellows and faculty were significantly more likely to have reported consulting with, meeting with, and planning treatment with a behavioral health provider during residency, and more often reported that their continuity clinic experience prepared them for collaborating with behavioral health providers, yet only somewhat more often believed that the overall residency training prepared them for handling behavioral health issues in their current practice.

Allison and colleagues[27] proposed that the future goals included expansion of behavioral health care for the many identified mothers, children, and adolescents within primary care. Ideally, patients who screen positive would benefit from assessments for safety, together with brief interventions and referral for ongoing care within the medical home. We have had great success with this through the support of a licensed certified social worker (CSW) embedded in our clinic. The mental health burden, however, remains high and calls for expansion of these services. Other innovative approaches we are piloting to address this need include having psychiatry residents in our clinic. Senior residents trained in psychiatry, pediatrics, and child psychiatry spend time each week in primary care to provide support in diagnosis and brief interventions. This model has the added benefit of educating our pediatric residents with resident peers supported by a child psychiatry attending. With continued effort to increase access to CSW and child psychiatry providers, in addition to the IBH Collaborative support in evidence-based improvement initiatives, we hope to strengthen and expand the integration of behavioral health into our primary care office to provide optimal and comprehensive care.

A review of IBH in pediatric care[28] demonstrated that continued integration includes (1) training medical and behavioral staff to broaden skills, (2) implementing universal behavioral health screening, (3) developing a tiered approach to treatment based on the identified needs of the patients, (4) utilizing care coordination and management, and (5) involving outside consultation to psychiatry when appropriate for medication management, level of care consultation, and/or inpatient/hospitalization consultation.

The opportunity clearly exists for child psychiatrists and psychologists with specialty training in pediatric primary care to provide integrated behavioral health services to help close the access gap. The ability of children and adolescents to have accessible, high-quality, evidence-based, prompt, and effective treatments to address behavioral health needs can be accomplished in pediatric primary care settings, using integrated behavioral health services.

RESIDENCY PROGRAM IN PEDIATRICS IN INDIA

In India, we have well-established PG courses for pediatrics: Medical Doctor (MD) and Diplomate in National Board (DNB) in Pediatrics. There are also Diplomas in Child Health (DCH). As yet we do not have any courses for PG in Adolescent Medicine/Pediatrics. Nearly 2000 seats for PG degree (MD and DNB) courses are available in teaching institutions, including medical colleges and hospitals. MD and DCH programs are accredited to a university, and DNB programs are accredited to National Board of Examination. A candidate possessing an MD degree can also appear for DNB for an additional qualification. However, this is not mandatory.

Successful candidates are registered as pediatricians by the Medical Council of India or state medical councils and they can practice as pediatricians. In most states, this registration is to be renewed every 5 years, with some states having made it mandatory for certain amount of continuing medical education credit hours and some states having no mandatory credit hours required for renewal of registration. Many of these new pediatricians also become members of IAP, which now has 33,000+ members. IAP offers a 1-year Fellowship in Developmental and Behavioral Pediatrics for candidates having MD/DNB in pediatrics. Various options are summarized in **Box 1**.

India has a well-established system of selection of students for undergraduate and PG medical courses. A central examination body conducts an entrance examination every year and the national medical counseling committee supervises the distribution of seats in nearly 530 medical colleges and teaching institutions every year.

A candidate should complete a 4.5-year graduation course (MBBS) and 1-year mandatory internship to become eligible for a PG course. The PG courses are regular full-time courses in which a candidate must work for 3 years in a hospital attached to a medical college or to NBE [National Board of Examination]. The teaching and training programs in these PG courses follow the curriculum prescribed by the Medical Council of India and the same is approved with minor modifications (if any) by the various universities and NBE. The exit examination is conducted and supervised by the

---

Box 1
After finishing the postgraduate (PG) program in pediatrics, most pediatricians follow one of the following paths

1. Most of them start a stand-alone clinic where they set up immunization services and outpatient department consultation. For indoor admissions, they tie up with the nursing homes nearby, which have facilities for pediatric beds.

2. Some set up hospitals and nursing homes from family money or bank loans.

3. Some of them come from families in which one or both parents already have a hospital or nursing home. So, they join this readymade infrastructure as pediatricians.

4. In the metro cities, there are a large number of multispecialty corporate hospitals where they join the pediatric department. Many of them have DNB students and research facilities.

5. Many medical colleges and hospitals have a residency scheme that provides for 3-year residency, and the candidate works as a senior resident and participates in patient care, teaching, and training activities.

6. After 1 year of working as a senior resident, one becomes eligible to work as an assistant professor in a medical college or a PG teaching institution. Some institutions require 3 years' experience for eligibility for the post of assistant professor.

7. Some state and central government hospitals also employ pediatricians who have 3 years' experience of working in a hospital as nonteaching specialists.

8. In the past, some who liked teaching or looking after the poor patients free of charge could join as an honorary pediatrician in government medical colleges with a nominal honorarium. Most of us benefited from such teachers, as they brought with them the rich expertise of clinical cases in the private sector, which we were not used to in the medical college patients. But for the past many years, this has been discontinued and medical colleges now have only full-time teachers.

universities and NBE. This includes 4 theory papers of 3 hours' duration and a practical skill assessment examination conducted by internal (same institution) and external examiners.

The 3-year curriculum includes a thesis or dissertation also to make the candidate competent in research methods. These PG students work in all the sections and units of the Department of Pediatrics including outpatient clinics, special clinics, indoor wards, neonatology wards, and emergency and critical care services. Some institutions have a rotation of PG students in other specialty departments, such as cardiology, neurology, pediatric surgery, physical medicine, and rehabilitation. The MCI [Medical Council of India] curriculum prescribes a rotation to community services also.

The PG curriculum in pediatrics (by MCI) includes behavioral health and psychiatric conditions also.[29] However, it does not instruct for rotation to psychiatry services. The competency-based curriculum includes (in syllabus) the behavioral and developmental disorders as a major heading. These disorders include rumination, pica, enuresis, encopresis, sleep disorders, habit disorders, breath-holding spells, anxiety disorders, mood disorders, temper tantrums, attention deficit hyperactivity disorders, and autism.

Behavioral health (BH) topics are discussed in PG teaching/training programs and one or more topics also become part of theory examination. However, BH topics are not considered as must-know areas. It is not common to find a teaching faculty in the Department of Pediatrics having a special interest in BH (and mental health) issues. In medical conferences also these topics hardly get prominence.

We could not find a study documenting reasons for the low priority given to BH. The probable reasons can be the very busy schedule of pediatricians for physical diseases, lack of expertise in the pediatrics faculty, lack of facilities (and mental health professionals, psychologists, counselors, and child psychiatrists) for mental health issues in country, lack of importance given to BH problems by the community, and poor financial reimbursement for the time spent in treating BH problems.

With the global epidemic of noncommunicable diseases (NCDs), the World Health Organization has identified 4 NCDs for global intervention: cardiovascular diseases, diabetes, chronic pulmonary diseases, and cancer; a healthy lifestyle is the key factor in disease prevention. A healthy lifestyle and equilibrium of mind, body, and spirit are the key factors of Ayurveda, and are being incorporated by allopathic doctors in the practice of modern medicine.[30,31]

Therefore, IBH will be very much accepted in Indian training of allopathic medicine. In fact, the authors would subsequently like to conduct a pilot program for implementation of IBH in pediatric residency training in some centers in India.

PUBLIC HEALTH SCENARIO

The Government of India has been implementing a strong maternal and child health and immunization program since the 1970s that was considered an essential component in the medical and nursing curricula. The child health and immunization programs were included in pediatric education so that the future doctors are oriented to the national programs and help implement when they join government service or undertake private practice. The national adolescent reproductive and sexual health program was launched in 2005 and later upgraded as the national adolescent health program in 2014[9] with a broad-based package that prominently included mental health and well-being, prevention of noncommunicable diseases (as the risk behaviors originate in this age group) and violence, in addition to nutrition, sexual and reproductive health, and substance use. In tune with the national program, adolescent health is being included in pediatric undergraduate and PG education. IBH would complement the national efforts for comprehensive improvement of the child and adolescent health and augment the competencies of pediatric residents.

HOW CULTURE COULD IMPACT INTEGRATED BEHAVIORAL HEALTH IN PEDIATRIC PRACTICE IN INDIA

For Indian culture, IBH is not a new concept. Ayurveda medicine ("Ayurveda" for short) is one of the world's oldest holistic ("whole-body") healing systems. It was developed more than 5000 years ago in India. Ayurveda defines health as Swasthya, which actually means "being contented in ones' natural state of inner harmony": one is considered as healthy when body, mind, and spirit are in the state of equilibrium, comfort, and bliss. The word Ayurveda is derived from 2 Sanskrit words: *Ayur* means *life* and *Veda* means *science,* so Ayurveda means *science of life.* Ayurvedic medicine seeks to create a healthy strong body through a series of diet, exercise, and lifestyle practices, including sleep and mindful living.

India has a rich cultural heritage, and most people follow one or the other religion. A large proportion of people would consider disease and disability (physical and mental) a curse of God for some past acts. Although, people do take care of physical diseases and, to some extent, BH issues also. However, it is yet to become a common practice to take professional help for BH issues. Several BH issues in children are considered part of their personality and are ignored; however, facilities are lacking for appropriate management even when it is diagnosed.

There are very few child psychiatrists in country and only 2 to 3 institutions offer Doctorate of Medicine (DM) courses in child psychiatry. Similarly, there is a lack of clinical psychologists, psychiatry or mental health social workers, and nurse counselors. However, more people now understand the significance of these professionals. There is a long way to go to even think of having an adequate number of health care professionals providing BH and mental health services as required in this country of 1.3 billion people. The number of psychiatrists in India are too few; there are 0.75 psychiatrists per 100,000 people,[32] as against the desired 3 psychiatrists per 100,000 people.

People still take refuge in traditional healers for severe BH issues and, at times, these healers relate the BH (and mental health) issues to evil spirits. Such things prevent the access to modern treatment and very often cause significant delay in treatment. Legislation, including the Mental Healthcare Act 2017,[33] Protection of Children from Sexual Offences (Amendment) Act 2019,[34] and Juvenile Justice (Care and Protection of Children) Act 2015,[35] has provisions for adequate protection for children facing difficulties. Their implementation does not reach to all the needed children. Much needs to be done for providing social security to those who require it the most.

We are hopeful that when we begin finding and treating BH issues, society will welcome it and gradually the appropriate agencies will also provide the required care and support.

INTEGRATING BEHAVIORAL HEALTH IN PEDIATRIC RESIDENCY IN INDIA

Although currently there is no DM or MD program for Developmental Pediatrics or BH issues, the IAP offers a Fellowship in Developmental and Behavioral Pediatrics. However, the focus on BH is inadequate. Many pediatricians are now focusing on developmental pediatrics and they are quite sensitized to the mental health issues, such as learning disabilities and autism spectrum disorder, they can be motivated to take up other issues of BH also.

Currently the demand for such professionals is comparatively much lower than that for professionals for physical diseases. However, as the small family norm is becoming popular, parents explore all the avenues for management of BH issues. As pediatricians become confident in managing these children, the services will certainly improve. More and more pediatricians are likely to join this field (**Box 2**).

COLLABORATION: HOW INTEGRATED BEHAVIORAL HEALTH IN PEDIATRIC RESIDENCY PROGRAMS FOSTERS COLLABORATION WITHIN THE PRACTICE, COMMUNITY, NATIONALLY, AND INTERNATIONALLY

We also suggest the following for better training of pediatrics trainees in BH issues.

1. Advocacy efforts with heads of the departments of pediatrics to give importance to BH
2. Collaboration with psychiatry and physical medicine and rehabilitation departments
3. Collaborations of academic organizations (IAP, psychiatry associations, psychologist and counselors' associations)
4. Collaboration with organizations working in the disability sector
5. Developing and validating screening tools for BH
6. Making virtual self-learning training resources
7. Multispecialty task force/group to steer this movement
8. Documenting the success stories from leading institutions

Box 2
Ideas of how integrated behavioral health (IBH) could be incorporated into residency training programs in India

1. The new curriculum has included broadly most behavioral/mental health disorders in the syllabus for MD Pediatrics. However, as mentioned earlier too, the real focus on these topics is lacking during the training for MD Pediatrics. We suggest the following for dealing with behavioral health (BH) issues in pediatrics training. The well child visits should be promoted to include the screening of BH issues, and the anticipatory guidance of parents and adolescents regarding BH issues.

2. Advocacy efforts are needed for streamlining the postgraduate (PG) training programs to include BH issues and for including BH cases in the log book for PG students.

3. Prepare detailed curriculum and identify the competencies for dealing with children up to 18 years of age with BH issues.

4. Preparing and disseminating teaching training aids for BH issues.

5. Promoting BH in pediatrics with the help of departments of psychiatry, physical medicine and rehabilitation, and medical social workers.

6. Promoting the incorporation of BH services in the facilities for developmental pediatrics.

7. Advocating BH screening in a national program for screening of children and adolescents for common deficiency diseases, disability, and developmental disorders, also known as Rashtriya Bal Swasthya Karyakram.

8. Empowering school teachers in recognizing and referring of children and adolescents having BH issues.

9. Expand the understanding of behavioral determinants of child and adolescent health and development so that pediatric residents could work in collaboration with parents and families for promotion of health and development of children and adolescents.

9. Testing the change ideas and piloting the solutions
10. Recognition (at various levels) of professionals working in BH fields

CLINICS CARE POINTS

- Behaviour health issues are important in Pediatrics practice.
- Behaviour health should be included in the undergraduate and postgraduate (Pediatrics) curriculum. Professional associations of Pediatrics and Mental Health should jointly support this.
- The residents should be trained to recognise and treat behaviour health issues in children in a timely manner.

DISCLOSURE

The authors have nothing to disclose related to this article. No commercial entity has helped in preparation of this article.

REFERENCES

1. Kaur R, Vinnakota A, Panigrahi S, et al. A descriptive study on behavioral and emotional problems in orphans and other vulnerable children staying in institutional homes. Indian J Psychol Med 2018;40(2):161–8.
2. Jaisoorya T, Beena K, Beena M, et al. Prevalence and correlates of alcohol use among adolescents attending school in Kerala, India. Drug Alcohol Rev 2016;35(5):523–9.
3. Bagchi NN, Ganguly S, Pal S, et al. A study on smoking and associated psychosocial factors among adolescent students in Kolkata, India. Indian J Public Health 2014;58(1):50.
4. Sahu M, Gandhi S, Sharma MK. Mobile phone addiction among children and adolescents: a systematic review. J Addict Nurs 2019;30(4):261–8.
5. Malhotra S, Patra BN. Prevalence of child and adolescent psychiatric disorders in India: a systematic review and meta-analysis. Child Adolesc Psychiatry Ment Health 2014;8(1):22.
6. Sunitha S, Gururaj G. Health behaviours & problems among young people in India: Cause for concern & call for action. Indian J Med Res 2014;140(2):185.
7. T Jacob John IAP policy on age of children for pediatric care. Indian Pediatr 1999;36:461–3.
8. Bhave Swati Y. Presidential address XXXVII National Conference of the Indian Academy of Pediatrics Jan 27 2000. Indian Pediatr 2000;37:249–54.
9. RKSK Strategy Handbook. National Health Mission. Ministry of Health and Family Welfare. New Delhi: Government of India. Available at: https://nhm.gov.in/images/pdf/programmes/RKSK/RKSK_Strategy_Handbook.pdf. Accessed September 28, 2020.
10. Medical Council of India, Competency based Undergraduate curriculum for the Indian Medical Graduate, 2018. Vol. 1. Available at https://www.nmc.org.in/wp-content/uploads/2020/01/UG-Curriculum-Vol-II.pdf. Accessed March 21, 2021.
11. US Department of Health and Human Services. Mental health: a report of the Surgeon General—executive summary. Rockville (MD): US Department of Health and Human Services, Substance Abuse and Mental Health Services Administration, Center for Mental Health Services, National Institutes of Health, National Institute of Mental Health; 1999.

12. New Freedom Commission on Mental Health. Achieving the promise: transforming mental health care in America: final report. Rockville (MD): US Department of Health and Human Services; 2003. DHHS publication No. SMA-03-3832.

13. Kelleher KJ, McInerny TK, Gardner WP, et al. Increasing identification of psychosocial problems: 1979-1996. Pediatrics 2000;105(6):1313–21.

14. Costello EJ, Edelbrock C, Costello AJ, et al. Psychopathology in pediatric primary care: the new hidden morbidity. Pediatrics 1988;82(3 Pt 2):415–24.

15. Costello EJ, Shugart MA. Above and below the threshold: severity of psychiatric symptoms and functional impairment in a pediatric sample. Pediatrics 1992; 90(3):359–68.

16. Guevara JP, Greenbaum PE, Shera D, et al. Survey of mental health consultation and referral among primary care pediatricians. Acad Pediatr 2009;9(2):123–7.

17. Schroeder CS. Psychologists and pediatricians in collaborative practice. In: Resnick RJ, Rozensky RH, editors. Health psychology through the life span: practice and research opportunities. Washington, DC: American Psychological Association; 1996. p. 109–31.

18. Perrin EC. Collaboration in pediatric primary care: a pediatrician's view. J Pediatr Psychol 1999;24(5):453–8.

19. Accreditation Council for Graduate Medical Education. [November 12, 2008] Program requirements for residency education in pediatrics. 2007. Available at: http://www.acgme.org/acWebsite/downloads/RRC_prog_Req/320_pediatrics_07012007.pdf. Accessed July 25, 2020.

20. Kittredge D, Baldwin CD, Bar-on ME, et al. [11/12/08] APA educational guidelines for pediatric residency. 2004. Available at: http://www.ambpeds.org/egweb. Accessed July 25, 2020.

21. Kelleher KJ, Campo JV, Gardner WP. Management of pediatric mental disorders in primary care:where are we now and where are we going? Curr Opin Pediatr 2006;18(6):649–53.

22. American Academy of Pediatrics. The future of pediatric education II. Organizing pediatric education to meet the needs of infants, children, adolescents, and young adults in the 21st century. A collaborative project of the pediatric community. Pediatrics 2000;105(1 Pt 2):157–212.

23. American Academy of Pediatrics (Committee on Psychosocial Aspects of Child and Family H. The new morbidity revisited: a renewed commitment to the psychosocial aspects of pediatric care. Pediatr Nov 2001;108(5):1227–30.

24. American Academy of Pediatrics. [11/14/2008] Improving Mental Health in Primary Care Through Access, Collaboration, and Training. Available at: http://www.aap.org/mentalhealth/docs/IMPACT%20Fact %20Sheet.pdf. 2006. Accessed July 25, 2020.

25. Health Committee on Health Care Access and Economics Task Force on Mental American Academy of Child and Adolescent Psychiatry and Financial Barriers to Access and Collaboration Improving Mental Health Services in Primary Care: Reducing Administrative and Economics Task Force on Mental American Academy of Child and Adolescent Psychiatry and Financial Barriers to Access and Collaboration Improving Mental Health Services in Primary Care. Pediatrics 2009;123:1248–51. Available at: http://www.pediatrics.org/cgi/content/full/123/4/1248.

26. Garfunkel LC, Pisani AR, leRoux P, et al. Siegel educating residents in behavioral health care and collaboration: comparison of conventional and integrated training models. Acad Med 2011;86(2):174–9.

27. Heinly A, Bogus E, Golova N, et al. Pediatric Primary Care and Integrated Behavioral Health. R I Med J 2018;101(10):32-34.
28. Njoroge WFM, Hostutler CA, Schwartz BS, et al. Integrated behavioral health in pediatric primary care. Curr Psychiatry Rep 2016;18:106.
29. Medical Council of India. Guidelines for competency based postgraduate training programme for MD in paediatrics. Available at: https://www.mciindia.org/CMS/wp-content/uploads/2019/09/MD-Pediatrics.pdf. Accessed July 25, 2020.
30. Lele Dr RD – Ayurveda and modern medicine. 1986 . Body and Mind Chapter 12 : 267-280 Published by Bharatiya Vidya Bhavan, Mumbai Printed by R. Raman at Inland printers Mumbai.
31. Mrunal R. Shenwai, Kirti N. Tare: Integrated Approach Towards Holistic Health: Current Trends and Future Scope IJCRR Section: General Science Sci. Journal Impact Factor 4.016 ICV: 71.54
32. Garg K, Kumar CN, Chandra PS. Number of psychiatrists in India: baby steps forward, but a long way to go. Indian J Psychiatry 2019;61(1):104.
33. The Mental Healthcare Act 2017. Ministry of Law and Justice, Government of India. Available at: https://www.prsindia.org/uploads/media/Mental%20Health/Mental%20Healthcare%20Act,%202017.pdf. Accessed September 28, 2020.
34. Protection of Children from Sexual Offences (Amendment) Act 2019. Available at: https://www.prsindia.org/sites/default/files/bill_files/Protection%20of%20Children%20from%20Sexual%20Offences%20%28Amendment%29%20Act%2C%202019.pdf. Accessed September 28, 2020.
35. Juvenile Justice (Care and Protection of Children) Act 2015. Available at: http://cara.nic.in/PDF/JJ%20act%202015.pdf. Accessed September 28, 2020.

Integrated Behavioral Health in Pediatric Subspecialty Clinics

Ethel Clemente, MD[a],*, Gordon Liu, BA[b],
Maria Demma Cabral, MD[a]

KEYWORDS

• Pediatric subspecialty • Chronic illness • Diabetes • Asthma • Congenital heart

KEY POINTS

• One in 4 youth live with a chronic condition in the United States and often require complex medical care.
• Mental and behavioral health concerns are common in pediatric patients with chronic illnesses.
• Health care providers from subspecialty practices recognize the need for provision of comprehensive care, including integrated behavioral health.
• Youth with certain chronic conditions, such as diabetes, asthma, congenital heart disease, cancer, and cystic fibrosis, and their families benefit from behavioral interventions that allow successful transition to adulthood.

INTRODUCTION

With advancements in medical care and improved treatment of life-threatening illnesses, the burden of disease has shifted from acute illnesses to chronic conditions. It is estimated that as many as 25% of the pediatric population is affected by a chronic condition.[1] Because of the complexity of their care, most of these children and adolescents are seen in a subspecialty care setting, allowing more focused intervention. However, this focused attention to a specific organ system or disease makes specialty providers less attuned to identifying and appropriately addressing mental or behavioral health issues that are frequently associated with chronic illnesses.[2,3] Behavior and mental health concerns are common in pediatric patients with chronic illnesses,[4–6] but these concerns are likely not addressed during regular visits to their

[a] Department of Pediatric and Adolescent Medicine, Western Michigan University, Homer Stryker M.D. School of Medicine, 1000 Oakland Drive, Kalamazoo, MI 49008-1284, USA;
[b] Western Michigan University, Homer Stryker M.D. School of Medicine, 1000 Oakland Drive, Kalamazoo, MI 49008-1284, USA
* Corresponding author.
E-mail address: ethel.clemente@med.wmich.edu

Pediatr Clin N Am 68 (2021) 633–649
https://doi.org/10.1016/j.pcl.2021.02.012
0031-3955/21/© 2021 Elsevier Inc. All rights reserved.

subspecialists for the same reasons stated earlier, which poses a problem because these children and adolescents with comorbid behavior and mental health issues are more likely to be nonadherent to treatment regimens, ultimately increasing morbidity and causing increased burden to caregivers and families. Most pediatric chronic conditions require frequent appointments to their specific subspecialties, thus patients and their families often consider their subspecialist as their main care providers. Taking into consideration the concept and principles of a patient-centered medical home,[7] subspecialty practices have started integrating behavioral health into the care they provide, allowing a more comprehensive but directed approach to the patient needs.

CHRONIC ILLNESS IN CHILDHOOD AND ADOLESCENCE

Pediatric chronic illness or medical condition has been variably defined to include any physical, psychological, or cognitive problem lasting more than 3 months that impairs functioning,[8] affecting the youth's typical activities, with some requiring hospital admissions and/or receiving health care at home with or without comprehensive medical care.[9] Similarly defined are children with special health care needs affecting their physical, developmental, emotional, and behavioral aspects of living, and this definition was expanded to reflect the need for appropriate program planning for health and related services.[10] The increasing survival rates of affected children and adolescents in the last 3 decades became possible because of early detection and availability of specialized care. Such has been evident in potentially fatal conditions such as complex congenital disorders, preterm birth, and cancer.[11]

An estimated 15 million children less than age 17 years in the United States have a chronic health condition, with numbers expected to increase with variable prevalence for specific conditions. Childhood asthma and diabetes are considered to be most common of the chronic diseases, with type 2 diabetes increasing in numbers likely from increasing obesity rates.[1,12] An interesting notion on epidemiologic shift and social ecology of childhood has been presented stating that potential risk factors, particularly in obesity, include childhood toxic stress, parental absence, and increased poor nutritional health with sedentary lifestyle and uptake of multimedia use in younger generations.[11,12]

The higher burden of a chronic medical condition, affecting not just the pediatric patients but also their caregivers, sets a precedence for psychosocial problems.[4,5] Anxiety and depression have been identified as occurring more often in this population.[13–16] Unpredictable and pervasive events, invasive and recurring procedures, fear of life-threatening situations and death, perceived loss of control over one's life, as well as peer rejection and social stigma are just some of the many potential triggers. Addressing mental illness and behavior concerns has been a long-standing gap in pediatric care, most especially in patients with existing chronic illnesses.

BEHAVIOR AND MENTAL CHALLENGES IN PEDIATRIC CHRONIC ILLNESS

Chronic illness in youth is a major source of significant stress and, in someone who does not have the appropriate coping skills, persistent unaddressed stress can lead to morbidity and mortality. Once diagnosed with a chronic condition, such as cancer or diabetes, the child and parent will soon realize the gravity of the lifelong illness that can bring about challenges and burdens to both the medical and psychological health domains. Another consideration is the stress brought about by an acute inciting event related to the chronic disease, such as respiratory infection in a poorly compliant asthmatic. Foreseen long-term pharmacologic treatments and adherence pose another level of difficulty that is sure to affect mental health, especially in the adolescence period.[12]

As many as 20% of American children meet criteria for a mental health problem, and less than a quarter of those identified receive specialty mental health treatment.[17,18] At present, there is an increasing acceptance of the importance of providing basic mental health care in the primary care setting. Both the American Academy of Pediatrics (AAP) and the American Academy of Child and Adolescent Psychiatry (AACAP) recommend that identifying and managing less complex problems should be initiated in primary care.

In 2009, the AAP published a policy statement that proposed competencies to improved knowledge and skills for system-based practice, targeting all levels of clinical experience.[19] The following year, AACAP also released a guide for collaborative mental health care with pediatric care providers.[20] However, despite these efforts, primary care providers continue to identify barriers that prevent appropriate delivery of mental health care. Horwitz and colleagues[21] surveyed randomly selected AAP members in 2004, and again in 2013, to identify these barriers and to assess change. The results showed fewer barriers identified in 2013, but still reported inadequate training, lack of confidence in counseling, as well as time constraints during clinic visits.[21] This finding shows that there is still a need for support for primary care providers, thus the emerging consensus on the benefits of providing integrated behavioral health (IBH). This process of integrated care involves the addition of behavioral health services into medical care practices. The goal is to provide care that not just addresses mental health issues such as anxiety, depression, or mood disorders but also to looks into health behaviors and the patients or families' capabilities to adapt to stressors that can affect physical and psychosocial response to acute and chronic conditions.[22,23]

Being a parent to a child with chronic illness demands time, patience, and understanding, which in turn potentially increases parental stress and promotes family conflict. Part of caring for children and adolescents with long-standing conditions entails parental influence in assisting their children to adapt and attain good quality of life. A recent Cochrane Review by Law and colleagues[24] investigated the different parental psychological interventions conducted in different study groups to identify which methods were useful in developing skills, with the aim of well-being improvement not only for the individual but the family unit as a whole. The investigators found that cognitive-behavior therapy (CBT) and problem-solving therapy (PST) had short-term improvement on parenting behavior for those with children with cancer, chronic pain, diabetes, and traumatic brain injury, and long-term improvement in the first 2 chronic conditions. When comparing parental mental health, there was improvement in parents of children with cancer and chronic pain, but not for parents of children with diabetes with PST but not with CBT. Other psychological interventions studied, such as family therapy, motivational interviewing, and multisystemic therapy, did not offer any benefits for parents.[24]

Emerging literature in understanding how people adapt to living with a chronic condition provides insight when addressing the needs of affected individuals. Most of those studied had found ways for positive adjustment toward the condition. Recognition and characterization of both risk and protective factors for adaptive functioning are key with potential integration of multifaceted contexts from an environmental, sociocultural, and biological standpoint.[25] Some disease conditions allow for application of a biopsychosocial model. Subsequent discussion focuses on the more common chronic illnesses in childhood: diabetes, asthma, congenital heart disease, pediatric cancer, and cystic fibrosis.

INTEGRATED BEHAVIORAL HEALTH AND DIABETES MELLITUS

Diabetes mellitus is one of the most common chronic conditions in childhood. Approximately 98,000 children less than the age of 15 years are diagnosed with type 1 diabetes mellitus (T1D) worldwide, with an overall annual increase rate of about 3%.[26] The increasing incidence of pediatric obesity and type 2 diabetes (T2D) is also a growing concern, with an estimated 5000 new cases per year in the United States.[27,28] Despite advancements in medicine technology, recent data show an increase in mean hemoglobin A1c levels among teens and early adults.[29]

The complexity and unique demands of diabetes self-management require constant support from a multidisciplinary team that provides comprehensive care. In pediatric patients, cognitive and developmental changes necessitate regular reassessment of their needs as they get older. The landscape of T1D care in pediatrics has dramatically changed after results of the Diabetes Control and Complications Trial showed fewer microvascular complications with tighter glycemic control using intensive insulin regimens.[30] Administration of medications several times a day; the need for frequent monitoring of blood glucose levels; as well as changes to lifestyle, diet, and everyday routine are what patients and families have to deal with on a regular basis. Like with other chronic pediatric conditions, living with diabetes becomes a burden that can put a significant toll on a child's and other family members' emotional and psychosocial well-being. Youth with diabetes have an increased risk of having anxiety and depression. They are also prone to having diabetes distress, a term coined to describe an emotional state when people with diabetes have feelings of stress, guilt, or denial, as a result of the burdens of diabetes management.[31,32] This condition then results in decreased adherence to their diabetes regimens, leading to poor glycemic control and health outcomes.

The American Diabetes Association (ADA) and the International Society of Pediatric and Adolescent Diabetes (ISPAD) recommend screening for psychosocial issues and stressors that can affect diabetes management on a regular basis, with timely and appropriate referral or participation of mental health professionals.[33,34] This recommendation stems from several years of research showing the positive impact of mental and behavioral health interventions in terms of glycemic control and quality of life. However, several barriers to screening have been identified, such as medical providers' low confidence to identify emotional burdens because of inadequate training, time constraints, limited access to mental health providers, and inadequate reimbursement.[35] Garvey and colleagues[36] report that, among endocrinologists caring for young adults transitioning from pediatric care, scenarios involving mental health issues posed the most significant barrier in clinical care management.

The role of mental and behavioral health providers in multidisciplinary teams caring for patients with diabetes has been well established. Their expertise in child development, understanding family dynamics, and providing not just interventions but also prevention strategies makes them an essential part of the diabetes care team. Behavioral intervention strategies have shown efficacy in improving behavioral, psychological, and glycemic outcomes in youth with T1D, with programs involving trained behavioral specialists having the most successful outcomes.[37] Common practices during diabetes visits every 3 months include educational interventions to promote adherence, such as blood glucose monitoring, insulin administration, as well as lifestyle modification. These interventions are task-directed instructions typically delivered by the diabetes provider or certified diabetes educators. A meta-analysis by Hood and colleagues[38] showed that combined interventions resulted in better glycemic control compared with interventions that focus on direct behavioral processes.

Combined interventions also focus on behavioral tasks, while including interventions that promote strategies for coping and problem solving. Coping skills training, family interventions, and multisystemic interventions are among the more-researched behavioral strategies used in T1D, and are based on behavioral theories such as social cognitive theory, family systems theory, and the social ecological model.[37] These interventions have shown positive effects, particularly when family is involved in the process.[39,40] Studies that used coping skills training had variable impacts on glycemic control but overall resulted in improved quality of life among youth with T1D and parents.[41,42]

Motivational interviewing is another tool that psychologists and trained providers can use that allows intrinsic motivation and promotion of positive behavioral changes.[37] Brief, tailored interventions incorporated during quarterly diabetes visits showed improved family involvement while decreasing family conflict, and prevented further worsening of glycemic control.[43] In a randomized controlled trial done by Serlachius and colleagues,[44] a cognitive behavioral intervention program did not show significant improvement in glycemic control but showed improved psychosocial well-being among participants.

In the ideal setting, mental and behavioral health providers are on site during diabetes clinics and fully integrated into each clinic visit. In reality, few diabetes clinics have ready access to psychologists or social workers trained to address psychosocial issues. As mentioned, these providers hold a unique position of rendering a service that can be used for prevention or intervention. Also, integrated care models show that integration of these services into practices promotes family engagement, reduces barriers to care, and allows mental health providers to reach more individuals and families compared with off-site referral systems.[45] Given this limitation, other methods of IBH screening and interventions have been explored. Several validated tools for screening and assessments are available and well suited for use in diabetes care settings.[46] Mulvaney and colleagues[47] investigated using a Web-based, self-guided behavioral intervention, with participants receiving training and guidance on coping and problem-solving skills. Other interventions have used technology such as text messaging for delivery of task reminders or motivational messages, smartphone applications, or games.[48,49]

INTEGRATED BEHAVIORAL HEALTH AND ASTHMA

Patients with chronic allergic disease often experience psychosocial stress and reduced quality of life, which in turn contribute to exacerbation of disease.[50] Although many caretakers indicate that mental health support would be beneficial, few of them received those services. In the United States, more than one-quarter of people with asthma are children, and poor disease control in particular is highly associated with increased symptoms of anxiety and depression.[51] Given the strong associations between chronic illness with mental health disorders, models that use IBH have the potential to significantly improve quality of life for children and their caregivers.[52]

Low adherence rates are a significant issue complicating the care of patients with asthma, ranging from 22% to 78% in some studies.[53] Various factors contribute to this poor adherence, including improper inhaled medical use, forgetfulness, social implications with peer bullying, parental concerns regarding side effects, and lack of family support. Furthermore, mental health disorders such as depression or anxiety often affect adherence, which in turn may exacerbate the underlying pathophysiology and lead to a cyclic pattern of worsening disease.[52,53]

Current models use a patient-centered care model that focuses on education, well-being, and proactive care to create an individualized care plan that allows for self-management of asthma.[54] These approaches are still being refined, and many have shown positive trends or some significance toward improving medication adherence and asthma morbidity. Studies using individual and group psychotherapy interventions such as CBT and family therapy have shown reduced symptomatic burden and improved asthma-related quality of life.[55] A small preliminary study showed promising results with the use of longitudinal CBT, finding improved quality of life, reduced panic symptoms, and decreased rescue inhaler use; however, it was emphasized that further research is required.[56] A later review examined the effects of family therapy in addition to traditional medical regimes, showing improvements in lung function and daily symptom burden.[57] However, the review was limited to only 2 randomized controlled trials examining these interventions, and only 1 controlled for the effects of increased attention on outcomes.

Motivational interviewing techniques have also been used to improve self-management, showing promise with regard to motivation to change and improved medication adherence. One study implemented motivational interviewing of inner-city African American adolescents and their caregivers, focusing on individual goals, motivators, and values to build self-responsibility, and in turn improve medication adherence.[58] These interventions were well accepted and perceived to be helpful, increasing motivation and readiness to adhere to medication regimes; however, more objective studies were required to evaluate true adherence levels.[58] Other studies featuring asthma education and skills training for disease management through exploration of basic disease information, triggers, roles of medications, and usage technique showed self-reported positive outcomes in children.[59]

Community-level interventions, such as those in school systems, used interactive group learning to normalize difficulties with self-management, which may be useful in school settings without adequate nursing staff. However, studies are conflicted on the effectiveness of education, with 1 finding that many caregivers and children understood medication rationale and regimens but continued to self-report low adherence numbers to daily maintenance and controller medication.[60] Other reviews have shown inconsistent results, with some showing increases in certain age ranges, whereas others showed no difference in knowledge and quality of life compared with controls following enrollment in education programs.[60] A Canadian study examining the use of an integrated care program found a modest improvement in inhaled corticosteroid adherence through self-reported and objective measures.[61] However, improved adherence by study participants did not result in better asthma control, although the study faced low patient participation. A combination of all of these different interventions may have significant implications for asthma control and medication adherence, but further studies are still needed.

Psychologists and other members of the pediatric care team can contribute to asthma care through the use of psychotherapy, psychophysiologic control interventions, lifestyle changes, management and education techniques, as well as broader-scoped interventions with family and school environments.[55] With further research into the different techniques and their associated efficacy, IBH has shown promise as a potential adjunct to traditional medical therapy in clinical practice, particularly in pediatric populations.

INTEGRATED BEHAVIORAL HEALTH AND CONGENITAL HEART DISEASE

Congenital heart disease (CHD), the most common birth defect, affects an estimated 1 in 100 live births annually in the United States[62] and its prevalence is expected to increase because of medical and surgical treatment advancements. One in 4 infants of these children have a critical CHD, such as coarctation of the aorta, hypoplastic left heart syndrome (HLHS), tetralogy of Fallot (TOF), and transposition of the great arteries (TGA), and usually require surgical interventions in the first year of life.[62,63] The type and severity of cardiac defect, timing of diagnosis, and designated treatment dictate outcomes and survival, with around 80% to 90% of affected children surviving into adulthood.[63] Three in 10 CHDs are found in those with a genetic syndrome such as Turner syndrome, Noonan syndrome, and Down syndrome.[64]

In 2010, there were 1.4 million adults living with CHD in the United States,[65] who have higher likelihood of experiencing physical and psychosocial challenges in their lifetime. At a young age, children with CHDs are in need and receipt of additional and specialized health and educational services compared with their typically developing peers without CHDs.[66,67] Data from the 2016 National Survey of Children's Health found 60% of children with current heart conditions (although it was not specified whether congenital, acquired, or other) had at least 1 special health care need, with 1 in 4 children needing or receiving behavioral, developmental, and emotional treatment, including counseling.[68] Razzaghi and colleagues[67] analyzed the representative sample from the National Health Interview Survey conducted from 1997 to 2011 and found that children with CHDs have increased likelihood of medical comorbidities such as asthma; developmental disabilities such as autism spectrum disorder, attention-deficit/hyperactivity disorder (ADHD), and speech/language disorders; and psychosocial indisposition such as school absence and limited physical activity participation. However, despite these identified difficulties, adolescents aged 12 to 17 years used health care services the least.[67]

Similar to other chronic health conditions, children and adolescents with CHD have higher rates of internalizing disorders such as anxiety and depression, externalizing disorders such as ADHD and substance use disorders, and other neuropsychological conditions.[69–72] Those diagnosed with severe cardiovascular disease have even higher chances for psychological and cognitive problems, possibly because of the presence of congenital brain and chromosomal anomalies or poor brain perfusion during surgery.[72] During pubertal neurohormonal changes, the genetic predisposition plus the stressful CHD experiences further increase the adolescents' risk for internalizing problems.[72] Although teens do not let their CHD define them, they are aware of their differences and challenges compared with their peers without CHD.[73] Children and adolescents with CHD identified their parents as the main source of information and the main discussant during doctor visits, and only a few can define their heart condition.[74] It is important to educate and involve the young patients about their conditions even before transitioning to adult care and to assist in them assuming responsibility for their own health care. Clinicians should not underestimate patients' needs in discussing psychosocial topics unrelated to their cardiovascular states and, often, they prefer not to be treated differently from their healthy peers.[74]

Given the longevity of CHD treatment and its health implications, parents were found to have poorer mental health caused by the chronic stress on top of financial and physical challenges that also affect home relationships.[75] In particular, maternal responsiveness is affected by psychological distress, mood disorders, and traumatic experiences.[75] Parental overprotection increased the children's risk for internalizing disorders.[72] Therefore, early identification of psychiatric symptoms, targeted psychological and psychosocial interventions, and prompt mental health referral if indicated benefit children and adolescents with CHD and their parents or caregivers. Health care providers should explore medical and nonmedical concerns from both the patient and parent and the caregiver, and provide adequate psychosocial support.

With scientific advancements, refinement of medical and surgical treatment approaches of the cardiac lesions has increased survival into the adult years and shifted the focus to attaining good quality of life. The guidelines put forth by the joint efforts of the American College of Cardiology (ACC) and the American Heart Association (AHA) recommend young adults to establish care at an adult CHD (ACHD) center to identify the necessity and type of long-term care required.[76] There is systemic and comprehensive need for effective transition from pediatric-centered to adult-oriented care. Transition must be purposefully planned to address not only the medical but also the psychosocial, educational, and vocational needs of these young persons.[77] Discussions about transitioning must occur in early adolescence with formal coordination between the pediatric and adult services and education on the implications of the cardiac condition, with eventual referral to an ACHD specialist. Parental involvement is encouraged, with their role ultimately changing to more of a secondary, supportive one.[77] In a study done by Flocco and colleagues,[78] the adolescents enrolled in a CHD transition care model had improved health perception with acquired knowledge of their cardiac conditions from structured education and reduction of pain and anxiety from working with a counselor or psychologist. With the vast recognition of the nonmedical or noncardiac concerns, such as employment, reproductive health, and mental wellness,[73,79,80] part of the ACC/AHA recommendations is to include psychosocial screening of individuals with CHD and the families in assessing for cognitive, mood, and psychiatric disorders.[76]

Despite established knowledge of the special health care needs of children with chronic disease, such as those with CHD, few specialized programs exist, with a lack of evidence-based guidelines in clinical implementation of nonpharmacologic modalities. A systematic review by Tesson and colleagues[81] studied psychological interventions for people affected by childhood-onset heart disease and found limited controlled trials for the study population. There were 4 studies specific for adolescents and adults with CHD and 5 studies for parents, particularly mothers of children with CHD. The parent-focused programs revealed some improvements in psychological outcomes, including parent-infant psychotherapy and a school-readiness program that correlated with improved maternal anxiety, coping, and family functioning. However, the investigators found poor quality of evidence and inconsistent efficacy resulting in no improvement in psychological outcomes from interventions conducted in adolescents and adults.[81] A 2013 Cochrane Review studied existing randomized controlled trials comparing the effectives of CBT, psychotherapy, and counseling in addressing depression in adolescents and adults with CHD, but found no eligible trials of such treatments.[82]

Psychological care should not be limited to the individuals living with CHD. With fetal diagnosis, early family counseling on expectations, treatment, and complications regarding the CHD must take place. Early detection puts the expectant parents in an emotional state leading to clinical depression, although lower maternal quality of life has been found if the CHD diagnosis was made after baby was born.[75,83,84] In the first study of parents with infants with HLHS, traumatic stress was apparent.[85] Mental health problems have also been described in relation to the cardiovascular surgery the child had undergone.[75] There is a recognizable need to address parental concerns and distress with provision of much-needed specific psychosocial and psychoeducational interventions such as skills-related training, but often parents receive such services in the hospital, particularly in the intensive care unit. However, ongoing assessment must occur even on subsequent outpatient follow-ups, and providers should consider improving adaptive coping skills and enhancing parenting abilities.[83,85]

In 1 retrospective study, the psychology records of 100 adults with CHD were reviewed. Most had complex CHDs, with repaired TOF as the most common type, followed by TGA. Patients sought psychological services for generalized and heart-related/health-related anxiety, depressed mood, and coping difficulties. Some had reported history of substance abuse. Psychotherapy was recommended to 87 patients, with most initiating treatment. Services offered include cognitive therapy, relaxation techniques, and communication skills training, and an average of 8 sessions were used over a period of time. Subjective documentation revealed significant improvement to near resolution of psychological distress that interfered with daily functioning. Although not representative of the general ACHD population, the study still highlighted the benefit of integrated psychological care.[86]

Psychocardiology is a new specialty in medicine, with application of psychology to better the lives of cardiac patients when experiencing mental health challenges.[87] Indications for referral of cardiac patients to a clinical psychologist include assistance with a difficult transition from pediatric to adult care, preparation for and adjustment to scheduled surgical procedures and the use of heart devices with use of relaxation and CBT, and especially adolescents coping with psychosocial problems with their peers.[88] Peer-to-peer support has been shown to be beneficial in patients with ACHD[88] and can be applied to younger children.

Provision of multidisciplinary family-centered psychosocial care should encompass pediatric and adult congenital cardiology, psychologists, social workers, and clinical nurse specialists. Integration of psychosocial services from assessment to treatment within a clinical setting promotes congenital heart health.[76,83] Beyond the medical and physical limitations of having a CHD, recognition of the discussed psychological outcomes is essential. Research must focus on establishing standardized treatment approaches with incorporation of psychologically primed care with universal adaptation in all cardiac specialty clinics. With increased survival into adulthood, persons with CHD deserve to live their lives fully.

INTEGRATED BEHAVIORAL HEALTH AND CHILDHOOD CANCER

In 2018, there was an estimated 15,500 children and adolescents diagnosed with cancer in the United States, and cancer is still the leading cause of death by disease after infancy in the pediatric age group.[89] Although still rare compared with the other chronic conditions previously discussed, childhood cancer instigates a significant impact because of the associated higher rate of morbidity and mortality. As medical management advances and more affected children survive, the scope of care expands to cancer survivors. The physical and emotional stress associated with oncologic conditions, at diagnosis, during active treatments, and all the way through survivorship or bereavement, renders affected children and their families at significant risk for psychosocial and mental health issues.

As such, this subspecialty has been most successful at accepting the importance of integrating behavioral health into clinical practice. In 2015, an interdisciplinary group of pediatric oncology psychosocial professionals developed evidence-based and consensus-based standards for psychosocial care for children with cancer as well as their families.[90] Through decades of research and practical applications, several psychosocial interventions have been proved to be effective in providing support and positive outcomes. CBT, problem-solving skills training, and family therapy are just some of the more widely used interventions, directed and tailored not just for patients but also for parents and other family members.[91] Eccleston and colleagues[92] conducted an updated systematic review on the effects of psychological interventions for parents of children and adolescents with chronic illness, including cancer, which showed improved adaptive parenting behavior and mental health.

However, as with other subspecialties, translating this to full fruition has been a challenge. Barriers to effective screening and intervention include limited staff and resources, insufficient training and knowledge of available tools and standards of care, time constraints for providers, and the added burden of additional visits for patients and families.[93] Availability of mental health providers in outpatient and inpatient settings is crucial for implementation but continues to be limited, particularly for smaller pediatric centers that may not have as much funding to support having mental health specialists regularly as part of their multidisciplinary teams. With the increasing use of technology to deliver and augment health care, there is growing evidence of the efficacy of technology-based interventions on improving health care behaviors and quality of life, as well as in alleviating emotional distress, although whether or not they are equivalent to face-to-face interactions is yet to be established.[94]

INTEGRATED BEHAVIORAL HEALTH AND CYSTIC FIBROSIS

Cystic fibrosis (CF) has evolved from a deadly pediatric disease to a lifelong chronic condition in adults, affecting nearly 70,000 individuals worldwide, nearly half of whom are in the pediatric population.[95] A major contributor to this increased survival and improved life expectancy has been the use of early diagnosis, new therapies, and comprehensive multidisciplinary care. Although these advancements have increased survival and facilitated its transition to a chronic disease, patients with CF have encountered high rates of depression, anxiety, and nonadherence, leading to significant lifelong impairment, particularly in pediatric populations.[96] Furthermore, the newer generation of treatment strategies comes with challenges, namely their complicated and time-consuming nature, resulting in low treatment adherence and suboptimal treatment outcomes.[97]

CF care centers have developed many methods for integrating behavioral health practices into the routine care of patients. In 2016, the Cystic Fibrosis Foundation (CFF) and European Cystic Fibrosis Society (ECFS) developed mental health guidelines for greater integration of behavioral health care for patients with CF and their families.[98] The widespread implementation of mental health coordinators through a grant from the CFF has yielded significant improvements in detection and awareness of mental health issues, which was welcomed by both patients and their families. These strategies are key to building strong, long-term patient-provider relationships, which are associated with improved adherence to treatment regimens.[99] A key focus was addressing nonadherence in a collaborative and empathetic manner, using motivational interviewing and involving both the patient and family in decision-making, each of which have been shown to improve adherence in chronic illnesses.

Despite these advances, many barriers remain in implementing these effective strategies. Insufficient social worker or behavioral health coordinator time, office space, perceived patient burden, and safe storage of data were identified by providers as the most significant barriers to screening for behavioral health issues.[98] Although the CFF provided funding nationally for CF clinics in the United States, difficulty remains in implementing the appropriate staff and policies to meet the diverse needs of patients. Although massive progress has been made in improving physical health, the aggregate effects of emotional and behavioral health cannot be understated.[100] The associated negative effects of mood disorders on treatment adherence and quality of life show an avenue through which IBH resources may improve comprehensive care in CF clinics.[101] Despite this, more studies are required to evaluate the long-term effects of conditions such as anxiety and depression on patient outcomes, which in turn may influence future treatment plans.

SUMMARY

Children and adolescents living with a chronic condition often experience mental and behavioral challenges as they transition into adulthood. With the complex care needed and frequent follow-up visits, pediatric subspecialists are often identified as the main health care providers. Pediatric subspecialty clinics recognize the role and importance of an IBH model with a multidisciplinary approach that promotes easy access to behavioral health screening, stress management, and important educational interventions. Established programs in childhood cancer and CF provide a template for the use of different psychological interventions as use in children and adolescents with diabetes, asthma, and CHD.

CLINICS CARE POINTS

- Mental and behavioral health interventions such as CBT, PST, coping skills training, and motivational interviewing have been shown to improve health outcomes and quality of life for youth with chronic conditions.

- Emerging data show that the use of technology such as telehealth visits or Web-based intervention strategies can potentially address the gap of limited mental health providers; however, further research is needed to assess whether these would provide equivalent efficacy compared with in-person interventions.

DISCLOSURE

The authors have nothing to disclose.

REFERENCES

1. Van Cleave J, Gortmaker SL, Perrin JM. Dynamics of obesity and chronic health conditions among children and youth. JAMA 2010;303(7):623–30.
2. Barlow JH, Ellard DR. The psychosocial well-being of children with chronic disease, their parents and siblings: An overview of the research evidence base. Child Care Health Dev 2006;32(1):19–31.
3. Secinti E, Thompson EJ, Richards M, et al. Research Review: Childhood chronic physical illness and adult emotional health – a systematic review and meta-analysis. J Child Psychol Psychiatry Allied Discip 2017;58(7):753–69.
4. Pinquart M, Shen Y. Behavior problems in children and adolescents with chronic physical illness: a meta-analysis. J Pediatr Psychol 2011;36(9). https://doi.org/10.1093/JPEPSY/JSR042.
5. Thabrew H, Stasiak K, Hetrick SE, et al. Psychological therapies for anxiety and depression in children and adolescents with long-term physical conditions. Cochrane Database Syst Rev 2018;2018(12). https://doi.org/10.1002/14651858.CD012488.pub2.
6. Kline-Simon AH, Weisner C, Sterling S. Point Prevalence of Co-Occurring Behavioral Health Conditions and Associated Chronic Disease Burden among Adolescents. J Am Acad Child Adolesc Psychiatry 2016;55(5):408–14.

7. Baird M, Blount A, Brungardt S, et al. Joint principles: integrating behavioral health care into the patient-centered medical home. Ann Fam Med 2014; 12(2):183–5.

8. Van Der Lee JH, Mokkink LB, Grootenhuis MA, et al. Definitions and measurement of chronic health conditions in childhood: A systematic review. J Am Med Assoc 2007;297(24):2741–51.

9. Mokkink LB, van der Lee JH, Grootenhuis MA, et al. Defining chronic diseases and health conditions in childhood (ages 0–18 years of age): National consensus in the Netherlands. Eur J Pediatr 2008;167:1441–7.

10. McPherson M, Arango P, Fox H, et al. A new definition of children with special health care needs. Pediatrics 1998;102(1 Pt 1):137–40.

11. Halfon N, Newacheck PW. Evolving notions of childhood chronic illness. JAMA 2010;303(7):665–6.

12. Compas BE, Jaser SS, Dunn MJ, et al. Coping with chronic illness in childhood and adolescence. Annu Rev Clin Psychol 2012;8:455–80.

13. Benton TD, Ifeagwu JA, Smith-Whitley K. Anxiety and depression in children and adolescents with sickle cell disease. Curr Psychiatry Rep 2007;9(2):114–21.

14. Dantzer C, Swendsen J, Maurice-Tison S, et al. Anxiety and depression in juvenile diabetes: A critical review. Clin Psychol Rev 2003;23(6):787–800.

15. Pinquart M, Shen Y. Depressive symptoms in children and adolescents with chronic physical illness: an updated meta-analysis. J Pediatr Psychol 2011; 36(4). https://doi.org/10.1093/JPEPSY/JSQ104.

16. Barker MM, Beresford B, Bland M, et al. Prevalence and incidence of anxiety and depression among children, adolescents, and young adults with life-limiting conditions: a systematic review and meta-analysis. JAMA Pediatr 2019. https://doi.org/10.1001/jamapediatrics.2019.1712.

17. Ginsburg S, Foster S. Strategies to support the integration of mental health into pediatric primary care. Issue paper. Natl Inst Heal Care Manag Found 2009;p. 6–7.

18. Martini R, Hilt R, Marx L, et al. Best principles for integration of child psychiatry into the pediatric health home. Am Acad Child Adolesc Psychiatry 2012;p. 3.

19. Coleman WL, Dobbins MI, Garner AS, et al. Policy statement - The future of pediatrics: Mental health competencies for pediatric primary care. Pediatrics 2009;124(1):410–21.

20. DeMaso D, Martini R, Sulik LF, et al. A guide to building collaborative mental health care partnerships in pediatric primary care. 2010;(June):1-27.

21. Horwitz SMC, Storfer-Isser A, Kerker BD, et al. Barriers to the identification and management of psychosocial problems: changes from 2004 to 2013. Acad Pediatr 2015;15(6):613–20.

22. Peek CJ, The National Integration Academy Council. Lexicon for Behavioral Health and Primary Care Integration; 2013.

23. Schwartz LA, Feudtner C. Providing integrated behavioral health services to patients with serious pediatric illness. JAMA Pediatr 2019. https://doi.org/10.1001/jamapediatrics.2019.1683.

24. Law E, Fisher E, Eccleston C, et al. Psychological interventions for parents of children and adolescents with chronic illness. Cochrane Database Syst Rev 2019;3(3):CD009660.

25. Stanton AL, Revenson TA, Tennen H. Health psychology: psychological adjustment to chronic disease. Annu Rev Psychol 2007;58:565–92.

26. Patterson CC, Karuranga S, Salpea P, et al. Worldwide estimates of incidence, prevalence and mortality of type 1 diabetes in children and adolescents: Results

from the International Diabetes Federation Diabetes Atlas, 9th edition. Diabetes Res Clin Pract 2019;157:107842.

27. Dabelea D, Mayer-Davis EJ, Saydah S, et al. Prevalence of type 1 and type 2 diabetes among children and adolescents from 2001 to 2009. JAMA 2014; 311(17):1778–86.

28. Nadeau KJ, Anderson BJ, Berg EG, et al. Youth-onset type 2 diabetes consensus report: Current status, challenges, and priorities. Diabetes Care 2016;39(9):1635–42.

29. Foster NC, Beck RW, Miller KM, et al. State of Type 1 Diabetes Management and Outcomes from the T1D Exchange in 2016-2018. Diabetes Technol Ther 2019; 21(2):66–72.

30. The Diabetes Control and Complications Trial Research Group, Nathan D, Genuth S, et al. The Effect of Intensive Treatment of Diabetes on the Development and Progression of Long-Term Complications in Insulin-Dependent Diabetes Mellitus. N Engl J Med 1993;329(14):977–86.

31. Reynolds KA, Helgeson VS. Children with Diabetes Compared to Peers: depressed? Distressed? Ann Behav Med 2012;42(1):29–41.

32. Kreider KE. Diabetes distress or major depressive disorder? a practical approach to diagnosing and treating psychological comorbidities of diabetes. Diabetes Ther 2017;8(1):1–7.

33. American Diabetes Association. 13. Children and Adolescents: Standards of Medical Care in Diabetes-2020. Diabetes Care 2020;43(January):S163–82.

34. Delamater AM, de Wit M, McDarby V, et al. ISPAD Clinical Practice Consensus Guidelines 2018: Psychological care of children and adolescents with type 1 diabetes. Pediatr Diabetes 2018;19(July):237–49.

35. Weitzman C, Wegner L, Blum NJ, et al. Promoting optimal development: Screening for behavioral and emotional problems. Pediatrics 2015;135(2): 384–95.

36. Garvey KC, Telo GH, Needleman JS, et al. Health care transition in young adults with type 1 diabetes: Perspectives of adult endocrinologists in the U.S. Diabetes Care 2016;39(2):190–7.

37. Hilliard ME, Powell PW, Anderson BJ. Evidence-based behavioral interventions to promote diabetes management in children, adolescents, and families. Am Psychol 2016;71(7):590–601.

38. Hood KK, Rohan JM, Peterson CM, et al. Interventions with adherence-promoting components in pediatric type 1 diabetes: Meta-analysis of their impact on glycemic control. Diabetes Care 2010;33(7):1658–64.

39. Ayling K, Brierley S, Johnson B, et al. Efficacy of theory-based interventions for young people with type 1 diabetes: A systematic review and meta-analysis. Br J Health Psychol 2015;20(2):428–46.

40. Feldman MA, Anderson LM, Shapiro JB, et al. Family-Based Interventions Targeting Improvements in Health and Family Outcomes of Children and Adolescents with Type 1 Diabetes: a Systematic Review. Curr Diab Rep 2018;18(3). https://doi.org/10.1007/s11892-018-0981-9.

41. Grey M, Boland EA, Davidson M, et al. Coping skills training for youth with diabetes mellitus has long-lasting effects on metabolic control and quality of life. J Pediatr 2000;137(1):107–13.

42. Grey M, Jaser SS, Whittemore R, et al. Coping skills training for parents of children with type 1 diabetes: 12-month outcomes. Nurs Res 2011;60(3):173–81.

43. Laffel LMB, Vangsness L, Connell A, et al. Impact of ambulatory, family-focused teamwork intervention on glycemic control in youth with type 1 diabetes. J Pediatr 2003;142(4):409–16.
44. Serlachius AS, Scratch SE, Northam EA, et al. A randomized controlled trial of cognitive behaviour therapy to improve glycaemic control and psychosocial wellbeing in adolescents with type 1 diabetes. J Health Psychol 2016;21(6):1157–69.
45. Njoroge WFM, Hostutler CA, Schwartz BS, et al. Integrated Behavioral Health in Pediatric Primary Care. Curr Psychiatry Rep 2016;18(12). https://doi.org/10.1007/s11920-016-0745-7.
46. Young-Hyman D, De Groot M, Hill-Briggs F, et al. Psychosocial care for people with diabetes: A position statement of the American diabetes association. Diabetes Care 2016;39(12):2126–40.
47. Mulvaney SA, Rothman RL, Wallston KA, et al. An internet-based program to improve self-management in adolescents with type 1 diabetes. Diabetes Care 2010;33(3):602–4.
48. Markowitz JT, Cousineau T, Franko DL, et al. Text messaging intervention for teens and young adults with diabetes. J Diabetes Sci Technol 2014;8(5):1029–34.
49. Herbert L, Owen V, Pascarella L, et al. Text message interventions for children and adolescents with type 1 diabetes: A systematic review. Diabetes Technol Ther 2013;15(5):362–70.
50. Oland AA, Booster GD, Bender BG. Integrated behavioral health care for management of stress in allergic diseases. Ann Allergy Asthma Immunol 2018;121(1):31–6. https://doi.org/10.1016/j.anai.2018.05.002.
51. Yeh GY, Horwitz R. Integrative Medicine for Respiratory Conditions: Asthma and Chronic Obstructive Pulmonary Disease. Med Clin North Am 2017;101(5):925–41.
52. Membride H. Mental health: early intervention and prevention in children and young people. Br J Nurs 2016;25(10):552–7.
53. George M, Bender B. New insights to improve treatment adherence in asthma and COPD. Patient Prefer Adherence 2019;13:1325–34.
54. George M. Integrative medicine is integral to providing patient-centered care. Ann Allergy Asthma Immunol 2015;114(4):261–4.
55. Ritz T, Meuret AE, Trueba AF, et al. Psychosocial factors and behavioral medicine interventions in asthma. J Consult Clin Psychol 2013;81(2):231–50.
56. Lehrer PM, Karavidas MK, Lu SE, et al. Psychological treatment of comorbid asthma and panic disorder: a pilot study. J Anxiety Disord 2008;22(4):671–83.
57. Yorke J, Shuldham C. Family therapy for chronic asthma in children. Cochrane Database Syst Rev 2005;2005(2):CD000089.
58. Riekert KA, Borrelli B, Bilderback A, et al. The development of a motivational interviewing intervention to promote medication adherence among inner-city, African-American adolescents with asthma. Patient Educ Couns 2011;82(1):117–22.
59. Mosnaim GS, Pappalardo AA, Resnick SE, et al. Behavioral Interventions to Improve Asthma Outcomes for Adolescents: A Systematic Review. J Allergy Clin Immunol Pract 2016;4(1):130–41.
60. McClure N, Seibert M, Johnson T, et al. Improving Asthma Management in the Elementary School Setting: An Education and Self-management Pilot Project. J Pediatr Nurs 2018;42:16–20.

61. Guénette L, Breton MC, Grégoire JP, et al. Effectiveness of an asthma integrated care program on asthma control and adherence to inhaled corticosteroids. J Asthma 2015;52(6):638–45.
62. Hoffman JL, Kaplan S. The incidence of congenital heart disease. J Am Coll Cardiol 2002;39(12):1890–900.
63. Oster ME, Lee KA, Honein MA, et al. Temporal trends in survival among infants with critical congenital heart defects. Pediatrics 2013;131(5):e1502–8.
64. Ko JM. Genetic syndromes associated with congenital heart disease. Korean Circ J 2015;45(5):357–61.
65. Gilboa SM, Devine OJ, Kucik JE, et al. Congenital heart defects in the United States: Estimating the magnitude of the affected population in 2010. Circulation 2016;134(2):101–9.
66. Riehle-Colarusso T, Autry A, Razzaghi H, et al. Congenital heart defects and receipt of special education services. Pediatrics 2015;136:496–504.
67. Razzaghi H, Oster M, Reefhuis J. Long-term outcomes in children with congenital heart disease: National Health Interview Survey. J Pediatr 2015;166:119–24.
68. Chen M, Riehle-Colarusso T, Yeung LF, et al. Children with heart conditions and their special health care needs — United States, 2016. MMWR Morb Mortal Wkly Rep 2018;67:1045–9.
69. Luyckx K, Rassart J, Goossens E, et al. Development and persistence of depressive symptoms in adolescents with CHD. Cardiol Young 2016;26(6):1115–22.
70. DeMaso DR, Calderon J, Taylor GA, et al. Psychiatric disorders in adolescents with single ventricle congenital heart disease. Pediatrics 2017;139(3):e20162241.
71. Marino BS, Lipkin PH, Newburger JW, et al. Neurodevelopmental outcomes in children with congenital heart disease: evaluation and management: a scientific statement from the American Heart Association. Circulation 2012;126(9):1143–72.
72. Karsdorp PA, Everaerd W, Kindt M, et al. Psychological and cognitive functioning in children and adolescents with congenital heart disease: a meta-analysis. J Pediatr Psychol 2007;32(5):527–41.
73. Shearer K, Rempel GR, Norris CM, et al. It's no big deal": adolescents with congenital heart disease. J Pediatr Nurs 2013;28(1):28–36.
74. Lesch W, Specht K, Lux A, et al. Disease-specific knowledge and information preferences of young patients with congenital heart disease. Cardiol Young 2014;24(2):321–30.
75. Kolaitis GA, Meentken MG, Utens EMWJ. Mental health problems in parents of children with congenital heart disease. Front Pediatr 2017;5:102.
76. Warnes CA, Williams RG, Bashore TM, et al. ACC/AHA 2008 guidelines for the management of adults with congenital heart disease: a report of the American College of Cardiology/American Heart Association Task Force on Practice Guidelines (writing committee to develop guidelines on the management of adults with congenital heart disease). Circulation 2008;118:2395–451.
77. Heery E, Sheehan AM, While AE, et al. Experiences and outcomes of transition from pediatric to adult health care services for young people with congenital heart disease: A systematic review. Congenit Heart Dis 2015;10(5):413–27.
78. Flocco SF, Dellafiore F, Caruso R, et al. Improving health perception through a transition care model for adolescents with congenital heart disease. J Cardiovasc Med (Hagerstown) 2019;20(4):253–60.

79. Canobbio MM. Health care issues facing adolescents with congenital heart disease. J Pediatr Nurs 2001;16(5):363–70.
80. Chong LSH, Fitzgerald DA, Craig JC, et al. Children's experiences of congenital heart disease: A systematic review of qualitative studies. Eur J Pediatr 2018; 177(3):319–36.
81. Tesson S, Butow PN, Sholler GF, et al. Psychological interventions for people affected by childhood-onset heart disease: A systematic review. Health Psychol 2019;38(2):151–61.
82. Lane DA, Millane TA, Lip GY. Psychological interventions for depression in adolescent and adult congenital heart disease. Cochrane Database Syst Rev 2013;(10):CD004372.
83. Kasparian NA, Winlaw DS, Sholler GF. Congenital heart health": how psychological care can make a difference. Med J Aust 2016;205(3):104–7.
84. Jackson AC, Frydenberg E, Liang RPT, et al. Familial impact and coping with child heart disease: a systematic review. Pediatr Cardiol 2015;36(4):695–712.
85. Cantwell-Bartl AM, Tibballs J. Psychosocial experiences of parents of infants with hypoplastic left heart syndrome in the PICU. Pediatr Crit Care Med 2013; 14(9):869–75.
86. Ferguson M, Kovacs AH. An integrated adult congenital heart disease psychology service. Congenit Heart Dis 2016;11(5):444–51.
87. Molinari E, Bellardita L, Compare A. Clinical psychology and heart disease. In: Molinari E, Compare A, Parati G, editors. Clinical psychology and heart disease. Milan: Springer-Verlag; 2006. p. 5–18.
88. Callus E, Pravettoni G. The role of clinical psychology and peer to peer support in the management of chronic medical conditions - A practical example with adults with congenital heart disease. Front Psychol 2018;9:731.
89. Ward E, DeSantis C, Robbins A, et al. Childhood and adolescent cancer statistics, 2014. CA Cancer J Clin 2014;64(2):83–103.
90. Wiener L, Kazak AE, Noll RB, et al. Standards for the psychosocial care of children with cancer and their families: an introduction to the special issue. Pediatr Blood Cancer 2015;62(Suppl 5):S419–24.
91. Steele AC, Mullins LL, Mullins AJ, et al. Psychosocial Interventions and Therapeutic Support as a Standard of Care in Pediatric Oncology. Pediatr Blood Cancer 2015;62:S585–618.
92. Eccleston C, Fisher E, Law E, et al. Psychological interventions for parents of children and adolescents with chronic illness. Cochrane Database Syst Rev 2015;2015(4). https://doi.org/10.1002/14651858.CD009660.pub3.
93. Wiener L, Devine KA, Thompson AL. Advances in pediatric psychooncology. Curr Opin Pediatr 2020;32(1):41–7.
94. Ramsey WA, Heidelberg RE, Gilbert AM, et al. eHealth and mHealth interventions in pediatric cancer: A systematic review of interventions across the cancer continuum. Psychooncology 2020;29(1):17–37.
95. Stephenson AL, Stanojevic S, Sykes J, et al. The changing epidemiology and demography of cystic fibrosis. Presse Med 2017;46(6 Pt 2):e87–95.
96. Samsel C, Ribeiro M, Ibeziako P, et al. Integrated Behavioral Health Care in Pediatric Subspecialty Clinics. Child Adolesc Psychiatr Clin N Am 2017;26(4): 785–94.
97. Faint NR, Staton JM, Stick SM, et al. Investigating self-efficacy, disease knowledge and adherence to treatment in adolescents with cystic fibrosis. J Paediatr Child Health 2017;53(5):488–93.

98. Quittner AL, Abbott J, Hussain S, et al. Integration of mental health screening and treatment into cystic fibrosis clinics: Evaluation of initial implementation in 84 programs across the United States [published online ahead of print, 2020 Jul 10]. Pediatr Pulmonol 2020. https://doi.org/10.1002/ppul.24949.
99. Riekert KA, Eakin MN, Bilderback A, et al. Opportunities for cystic fibrosis care teams to support treatment adherence. J Cyst Fibros 2015;14(1):142–8.
100. Mueller AE, Georgiopoulos AM, Reno KL, et al. Introduction to cystic fibrosis for mental health care coordinators and providers: collaborating to promote wellness. Health Soc Work 2020. https://doi.org/10.1093/hsw/hlaa009. hlaa009.
101. Quittner AL, Abbott J, Georgiopoulos AM, et al. International Committee on Mental Health in Cystic Fibrosis: Cystic Fibrosis Foundation and European Cystic Fibrosis Society consensus statements for screening and treating depression and anxiety. Thorax 2016;71(1):26–34.

Barriers for Ethnic Minorities and Low Socioeconomic Status Pediatric Patients for Behavioral Health Services and Benefits of an Integrated Behavioral Health Model

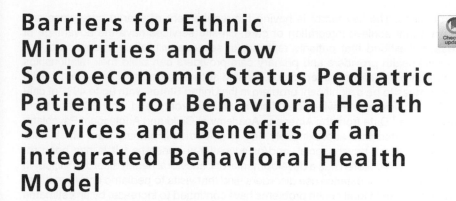

Cheryl Dickson, MD, MPH[a],*, Jessica Ramsay, MD[b],
Joshua VandeBurgh, MD[c]

KEYWORDS

- Ethnic minority populations • ADHD • Barriers to care • Low socioeconomic status
- Provider bias • Cultural competence • Cultural beliefs and stigma
- Integrated behavioral health

KEY POINTS

- Integrated behavioral health models within primary care settings can reduce key barriers to care experienced by ethnic minority and low socioeconomic status families.
- Disparities exist for black and Hispanic patients on multiple levels for behavioral and mental health services from early diagnosis to referrals and treatment.
- Provider awareness of barriers as well as training in cultural humility and implicit bias are key recommendations.

INTRODUCTION

The integrated behavioral health care (IBH) model in primary care settings has the potential to reduce many of the barriers for children and families who need to receive behavioral and mental health services.[1] The ideal model of IBH includes having behavioral health services on site in primary care settings but can also can include physically

[a] Associate Dean Health Equity and Community Affairs, 1000 Oakland Drive, Kalamazoo, MI 49009, USA; [b] Western Michigan University Homer Stryker MD School of Medicine, 1000 Oakland Drive, Kalamazoo, MI 49009, USA; [c] Department of Neurology, University of Minnesota Medical Center, 516 Delaware Street, SE 12-100 Phillips Wangensteen Building, Minneapolis, MN 55455, USA
* Corresponding author.
E-mail address: Cheryl.dickson@med.wmich.edu

Pediatr Clin N Am 68 (2021) 651–658
https://doi.org/10.1016/j.pcl.2021.02.013
0031-3955/21/Published by Elsevier Inc.

separate sites. The key factor is having the requirement of shared care plans and workflows that achieve integration of care. On-site services have the advantage of increased likelihood that patients referred for services will follow through and that behavioral health providers and primary care providers can build their relationships and skills through informal interactions. Limited access to pediatric behavioral health care continues to be a significant problem in the United States, with up to 40% of children and adolescents having identified mental disorders and only 30% of them receiving care.[1] Data from the American Academy of Child and Adolescent Psychiatry (AACAP) reported that approximately half of all pediatric primary care office visits involve behavioral, psychosocial, and/or educational concerns.[2] It is has been reported that 1 in 5 children has a developmental or behavioral health disorder, including mental health and substance use disorders, and that visits to pediatric emergency departments for behavioral health problems have continued to increase, by an estimated 47% during the years between 2003 and 2012.[3–5] Suicide is now the second leading cause of death among children 10 to 24 years old.[3] Even with this evident gap in services, a 2013 periodic survey of pediatricians revealed that less than 30% reported managing or comanaging any mental health condition other than attention-deficit/hyperactivity disorder (ADHD).[6,7] Because of the shortage of behavioral health providers, primary care providers provide most of the care for behavioral health and mental health problems and reported thinking that they lack the competence to provide these services adequately.[8]

Barriers to receiving behavioral and mental health services are discussed next.

BACKGROUND

There are multiple reasons that contribute to the barriers for children and adolescents in receiving needed behavioral health and mental services. Overall, barriers include decreased access to care because of transportation barriers, lack of insurance or nonacceptance of insurance by providers, behavioral health provider shortages, and stigma associated with cultural beliefs.[9,10] Average wait time for referrals for behavioral health services has been reported to be 6 months or longer.[11]

Barriers in Access to Care

Lack of medical home

These barriers are particularly evident in ethnic minority populations (African American and Hispanic) and low socioeconomic status (SES) families, where the need for behavioral health services is underscored by the lack of insurance, as well as lack of a primary medical home. A medical home as defined by the American Academy of Pediatrics (AAP) includes medical care of infants, children, and adolescents that is accessible, continuous, comprehensive, family centered, coordinated, compassionate, and culturally effective. Recommendations include that physicians should not only be well trained in primary care but that they should be able to facilitate all aspects of family care, and should be able to develop a partnership of mutual responsibility and trust.[12] Compared with white children, Hispanic and black children had a significantly decreased likelihood of having a medical home when they had an attention deficit disorder (eg, ADHD), developmental delay, or depression, and there were significant racial/ethnic disparities among children with special health care needs with mental disorders.[13]

Problems with providers

There are multiple barriers related to providers that limit access to behavioral health care. There is a lack of trained providers, especially in pediatric and early childhood mental health. This lack is exacerbated by long wait times and insufficient insurance payment for services, which further increases the barrier to care.[10] Poorer access to basic health services caused by poorer access to insurance[14,15] plays a role; however, reports in the literature reveal that minorities with insurance still have poorer access to care even after insurance status is taken into account.[16,17] The care when received for minorities and patients with low English proficiency has been reported to be of lower quality.[18] For example, although children may access care, they may not receive all the recommended services, such as desired anticipatory guidance or family-centered care, both of which are associated with early identification of developmental and behavioral concerns.[18] Even more concerning are reports that, even after adjusting for socio-demographic differences, minority children with developmental delays, such as autistic spectrum disorder (ASD), have less access to family-centered care (medical home) than white children, which is critical to identification screening and referral for services.[19]

Barriers for receiving care also include problems with diagnosis and service for behavioral disorders for ethnic minorities related to health provider bias and lack of cultural competence.[20,21] Racial, ethnic, and language disparities are reported in the diagnosis and treatment of early childhood developmental and behavioral disorders, such as ASD and ADHD. African American children and Latino children are less likely to be diagnosed with an ASD, and, when diagnosed, they are more likely to be diagnosed at older ages and with more severe symptoms.[22,23] The same holds true for diagnosis and treatment of ADHD, where African American and Latino children are less likely to be treated with a stimulant medication once diagnosed.[24,25] Disparities have also been reported in diagnosis and treatment of depression and mental health disorders at later ages,[26,27] with differences in the use of psychotropic medications[28] and referral to mental health services.[29]

These racial and ethnic disparities deserve increased attention given recent demographic trends. Census estimates indicate that the US population younger than 5 years will be 50% racial and ethnic minority (http://www,census.gov/newsroom/releases/archives/population/cb12-90.html[28]) and some states are now majority minority for young children (http://www.ncir.org/index.php/publications[29]).

Barriers related to cultural and health beliefs

Contributing to later detection and entry into behavioral and mental health services are varying cultural differences and health beliefs about child development and behavior among parents of African American and Latino children. Differing beliefs about when certain basic developmental milestones should be achieved are an example, as well as how important it is to talk to and read to young children.[30,31] Studies have reported and suggested that parental understandings of the limits of typical child behavior may have an impact on specific developmental behavioral problems, resulting in differing rates of mental health care use. For example, a large survey of parents of youths with mental health problems reported that African American, Asian/Pacific Islander, and Latino parents were less likely to view emotional behavioral problems as having a mental health basis.[29] Similar studies and surveys have shown that some ethnic minority families are more likely to attribute mental health symptoms to emotional or personality conditions and are less likely to agree with mental health professionals' labels of the conditions, and are less aware of the symptoms of common mental health disorders, including ADHD, leading to lower rates of mental health services use patterns.[24,29,32,33] In addition to differences in health beliefs, stigma surrounding use of mental health providers also may act as a barrier to accessing care. African American families reported higher likelihood of being embarrassed and fearing disapproval from family members with seeking mental health care, which is also related to belief that it is ineffective and unhelpful.[34] Latino parents are less likely to bring their children because of language and cross-cultural communication barriers. Cultural factors, as well as past historical factors related to health care experiences and medicine, have contributed to minority parents being less trustful of medicine. This lack of trust, combined with a lower likelihood of having a primary medical home, and the belief that there is less value in interacting with the health care and educational systems to receive care for developmental behavioral concerns, contributes to the barriers and ultimately the disparities seen in ethnic minority populations.[35]In many cases, these beliefs may be justified because evidence in the literature has shown that the mental health system does not perform as well for minority and other underserved families.[16,27]

DISCUSSION
Integrated Behavioral Health Model Benefits

Studies have shown that integration of behavioral health care models with on-site primary care services has improved pediatric access to care and treatment outcomes for common behavioral health disparities.[34,36,37] In the Integrated Behavioral Health Care in Pediatric Primary Care; Quality Improvement Project, described by Yogman and colleagues,[3] the investigators' data (although limited) indicated that the intervention of placing a licensed independent clinical social worker trained in child behavioral health care along with a parent partner/care coordinator in 3 primary care pediatric practices seemed to improve self-reported parental stress, family-centered care, and client satisfaction. Provider experience in the practice as a whole also improved. Reports of improvement in the practice included team development, family-centered care, and physician belief measures with efficiency and decreased burden in treating behavioral problems.[3]Studies have reported that ethnic minorities are more likely to report behavioral health concerns in the primary care setting and less likely to receive care in outpatient mental health settings[38,39]; therefore, provision of mental health services within primary care settings can be seen as a one of the ways to attempt to address disparities that ethnic minorities experience relative to mental health assessment, diagnosis, and treatment. The primary care setting offers an opportunity for patients with comprehensive physical, mental, and behavioral health problems to elucidate their concerns. On-site colocation of behavioral health services should be beneficial in providing improved entry for patients into care as well as follow-up appointments and treatment compliance with care plans.[40] Interface between behavioral health and medical personnel can lead to improved diagnosis, monitoring of medication side effects, and outcomes.[40] In addition, colocation may decrease stigma and discrimination while increasing opportunities for improved health.[41] Important considerations for reducing health disparities also include implementation, monitoring, and tracking of local, state, and national health policies; improving access to comprehensive integrated and patient-centered quality care; and promotion of culturally centered prevention and intervention approaches for vulnerable populations. Although there is an absence of strong evidence about the effectiveness of culturally centered integrated health care models to address health and mental health issues for ethnically and culturally diverse patients,[42] there are observations evident in the research literature that support the promise of improved relationship between patients and their experiences within health care settings and health care provider behaviors with awareness, training, and inclusion of cultural sensitivity.[21,42] Continued outreach, training, education, and recruitment of increased ethnic and cultural diversity in the health care and behavioral health care workforce is needed as well, which will add to reduction of disparities seen with health outcomes for ethnic minority patients.

SUMMARY

When considering future research directions, it is important consider previous challenges to conducting and researching interventions that eliminate disparities. Specific past challenges have included significant attrition in studies when working with disadvantaged populations, lack of availability of study personnel from the target community, unfamiliarity of institutional review boards with disparities interventions and community-based research, and lack of sustainability for successful interventions.[43] Looking toward the future, additional research is needed to clarify the mechanisms underlying various disparities in order for interventions to be successful. Differing mechanisms contributing to disparities will likely require unique interventions and implementation, as well as unique policy solutions.[16] A previous example given by researchers engaged in this work is a disparity that exists in part because of parental attitudes in a given community, in which case the intervention may need to be educational. However, if a disparity is driven by service availability to the community, a separate set of interventions directed toward developing and allocating resources may be needed.[16] Some research has indicated that the presence of an on-site mental health practitioner, in itself, is not sufficient to enhance practices related to common child and adolescent mental health problems.[7] This finding reinforces the assertion by Kataoka and colleagues[16] that there are multiple mechanisms for disparity, and additional research is needed into those mechanisms in order to determine adequate solutions. Further, when implementing interventions such as various integrated behavioral health models, it is important to analyze the efficacy of those interventions and their impacts on the community being served. In an article examining integrated behavioral health for Latino people, Manoleas[44] proposes a set of questions for future research. Although his article and proposal were specific to the Latino context, a modified set of questions may be instructive and critical to explore for other marginalized communities:

1. What is the effect of primary care and behavioral health integration on the current disparities in the use of behavioral health/mental services in the populations being served?
2. What effect does integration of primary care and behavioral health have on the psychiatric symptoms and other psychosocial issues of the patients being served?
3. How does integration of primary care and behavioral health affect other health outcomes, such as treatment adherence, chronic disease management, and the promotion of healthy behaviors? Many recommendations and research proposals are focused at the provider/clinic level. However, many disparities arise from larger systemic issues. Future research should be encouraged to examine larger systems-based interventions, including policy and regulatory change that may affect behavioral/mental health access for racial and ethnic minorities, and those of low economic social status. The authors specifically encourage working with professional societies, advocacy groups, and state agencies to effect systems-level change.[45]

CLINICS CARE POINTS

- Integration of behavioral health care models with on-site primary care services has been reported to improve pediatric access to care and treatment outcomes for common behavioral health disparities affecting ethnic minority families.

- On-site colocation of behavioral health services can be beneficial in several ways, including entry to care, follow-up, treatment compliance, and reduction of stigma and discrimination while improving opportunities for improved health.

DISCLOSURE

The authors have no disclosures.

REFERENCES

1. Njoroge WF, Hostutler CA, Schwartz BS, et al. Integrated Behavioral Health in Pediatric Primary Care. Curr Psychiatry Rep 2016;18(12):106.
2. Martini R, Hilt R, Marx L, et al. Best principles for integration of child psychiatry into the pediatric health home. Am Acad Child Adolesc Psychiatry 2012;2–13.
3. Yogman MW, Betjemann S, Sagaser A, et al. Integrated behavioral health care in pediatric primary care: a quality improvement project. Clin Pediatr (Phila) 2018; 57(4):461–70.
4. Mahajan P, Alpern ER, Grupp-Phelan J, et al. Epidemiology of psychiatric-related visits to emergency departments in a multicenter collaborative research pediatric network. Pediatr Emerg Care 2009;25(11):715–20. Available at: http://ovidsp. ovid.com/ovidweb.cgi?
T=JS&PAGE=reference&D=emed12&NEWS=N&AN=358038911.
5. Pittsenbarger ZE, Mannix R. Trends in pediatric visits to the emergency department for psychiatric illnesses. Acad Emerg Med 2014;21(1):25–30.
6. Green C, Storfer-Isser A, Stein REK, et al. Which Pediatricians Comanage Mental Health Conditions? Acad Pediatr 2017;17(5):479. Available at: http://www.ncbi. nlm.nih.gov/pubmed/28279638.
7. McCue Horwitz S, Storfer-Isser A, Kerker BD, et al. Do on-site mental health professionals change pediatricians' responses to children's mental health problems? Acad Pediatr 2016;16(7):676–83.
8. Power TJ, Mautone JA, Manz PH, et al. Managing attention-deficit/hyperactivity disorder in primary care: a systematic analysis of roles and challenges. Pediatrics 2008;121(1):e65–72. Available at: http://pediatrics.aappublications.org/cgi/ doi/10.1542/peds.2007-0383.
9. Benzer JK, Beehler S, Miller C, et al. Grounded theory of barriers and facilitators to mandated implementation of mental health care in the primary care setting. Depress Res Treat 2012;2012:1–11. Available at: http://www.hindawi.com/ journals/drt/2012/597157/.
10. Bishop TF, Press MJ, Keyhani S, et al. Acceptance of insurance by psychiatrists and the implications for access to mental health care. JAMA Psychiatry 2014; 71(2):176–81.
11. Grupp-Phelan J, Harman JS, Kelleher KJ. Trends in mental health and chronic condition visits by children presenting for care at U.S. emergency departments. Public Health Rep 2007;122(1):55–61.
12. Abuse C. American academy of pediatrics. Pediatrics 2001;107(2):437–41.
13. Park C, Tan X, Patel IB, et al. Racial health disparities among special health care needs children with mental disorders: Do medical homes cater to their needs? J Prim Care Community Health 2014;5(4):253.
14. Flores G, Abreu M, Tomany-Korman SC. Why Are Latinos the Most Uninsured Racial/Ethnic Group of US Children? A Community-Based Study of Risk Factors for and Consequences of Being an Uninsured Latino Child. Pediatrics 2006;

118(3):e730–40. Available at: http://pediatrics.aappublications.org/cgi/doi/10. 1542/peds.2005-2599.

15. Flores G, Lin H. Trends in racial/ethnic disparities in medical and oral health, access to care, and use of services in US children: has anything changed over the years? Int J Equity Health 2013;12(1):10.

16. Kataoka SH, Zhang L, Wells KB. Unmet need for mental health care among U.S. children: Variation by ethnicity and insurance status. Am J Psychiatry 2002; 159(9):1548.

17. Ngui EM, Flores G. Unmet Needs for Specialty, Dental, Mental, and Allied Health Care among Children with Special Health Care Needs: Are There Racial/Ethnic Disparities? J Health Care Poor Underserved 2007;18(4):931–49. Available at: http://muse.jhu.edu/content/crossref/journals/journal_of_health_care_for_the_ poor_and_underserved/v018/18.4ngui.html.

18. Guerrero A, Rodriguez M, Flores G. Disparities in Provider Elicitation of Parents' Developmental Concerns for US Children. Pediatrics 2011;128(5):901–9. Available at: www.pediatrics.org/cgi/doi/10.1542/peds.2011-0030. Accessed January 30, 2019.

19. Montes G, Halterman JS. White-black disparities in family-centered care among children with autism in the United States: Evidence from the NS-CSHCN 2005-2006. Acad Pediatr 2011;11(4):297–304.

20. Holden K, McGregor B, Thandi P, et al. Toward culturally centered integrative care for addressing mental health disparities among ethnic minorities. Psychol Serv 2014;11(4):357.

21. Malhotra K, Shim R, Baltrus P, et al. Racial/ethnic disparities in mental health service utilization among youth participating in negative externalizing behaviors. Ethn Dis 2015;25(2):123.

22. Mandell DS, Wiggins LD, Carpenter LA, et al. Racial/ethnic disparities in the identification of children with autism spectrum disorders. Am J Public Health 2009; 99(3):493–8.

23. Pedersen A, Pettygrove S, Meaney FJ, et al. Prevalence of Autism Spectrum Disorders in Hispanic and Non-Hispanic White Children. Pediatrics 2012;129(3): e629–35. Available at: http://pediatrics.aappublications.org/cgi/doi/10.1542/ peds.2011-1145.

24. Bussing R, Zima BT, Gary FA, et al. Barriers to detection, help-seeking, and service use for children with ADHD symptoms. J Behav Health Serv Res 2003;30(2): 176–89.

25. Pastor PN, Reuben CA. Racial and ethnic differences in ADHD and LD in young school-age children: Parental reports in the national health interview survey. Public Health Rep 2005;120(4):383–92.

26. Chabra A, Chávez GF, Harris ES. Mental illness in elementary-school-aged children. West J Med 1999;170(1):28–34. Available at: https://www.scopus.com/ inward/record.uri?eid=2-s2.0-0344958882&partnerID=40&md5=c4271cdae28f871691b31be2bd758460.

27. Zimmerman FJ. Social and economic determinants of disparities in professional help-seeking for child mental health problems: Evidence from a national sample. Health Serv Res 2005;40(5 Pt 1):1514–33.

28. Leslie LK, Weckerly J, Landsverk J, et al. Racial/ethnic differences in the use of psychotropic medication in high-risk children and adolescents. J Am Acad Child Adolesc Psychiatry 2003;42(12):1433.

29. Yeh M, McCabe K, Hough RL, et al. Why bother with beliefs? Examining relationships between race/ethnicity, parental beliefs about causes of child problems, and mental health service use. J Consult Clin Psychol 2005;73(5):800–7.
30. Pachter LM, Dworkin PH. Maternal expectations about normal child development in 4 cultural groups. Arch Pediatr Adolesc Med 1997;151(11):1144–50.
31. Bornstein MH, Cote LR. "Who Is Sitting Across From Me?" Immigrant Mothers' Knowledge of Parenting and Children's Development. Pediatrics 2004;114(5): e557–64. Available at: http://pediatrics.aappublications.org/cgi/doi/10.1542/peds.2004-0713.
32. Bussing R, Schoenberg NE, Perwien AR. Knowledge and information about ADHD: Evidence of cultural differences among African-American and white parents. Soc Sci Med 1998;46(7):919–28.
33. Guarnaccia PJ, Parra P. Ethnicity, social status, and families' experiences of caring for a mentally ill family member. Community Ment Health J 1996;32(3):243–60.
34. Richardson LA. Seeking and obtaining mental health services: What do parents expect? Arch Psychiatr Nurs 2001;15(5):223–31.
35. Rajakumar K, Thomas SB, Musa D, et al. Racial Differences in Parents' Distrust of Medicine and Research. Arch Pediatr Adolesc Med 2010;163(2):108–14.
36. Asarnow JR, Jaycox LH, Duan N, et al. Effectiveness of a quality improvement intervention for adolescent depression in primary care clinics: a randomized controlled trial. JAMA 2005;293(3):311–9.
37. Kolko DJ, Campo J, Kilbourne AM, et al. Collaborative care outcomes for pediatric behavioral health problems: a cluster randomized trial. Pediatrics 2014;133(4): e981–92. Available at: http://pediatrics.aappublications.org/cgi/doi/10.1542/peds.2013-2516.
38. Cooper LA, Gonzales JJ, Gallo JJ, et al. The Acceptability of Treatment for Depression among African-American, Hispanic, and White Primary Care Patients. Med Care 2003;41(4):479–89. Available at: http://www.jstor.org/stable/3767760.
39. Sentell T, Shumway M, Snowden L. Access to mental health treatment by English language proficiency and race/ethnicity. J Gen Intern Med 2007;22(Suppl 2):289.
40. Bauer AM, Azzone V, Goldman HH, et al. Implementation of collaborative depression management at community-based primary care clinics: an evaluation. Psychiatr Serv 2011;62(9). Available at: http://psychiatryonline.org/article.aspx?doi=10.1176/appi.ps.62.9.1047.
41. Aguirre J, Carrion VG. Integrated behavioral health services: A collaborative care model for pediatric patients in a low-income setting. Clin Pediatr (Phila) 2013; 52(12):1178–80.
42. Tucker CM, Herman KC, Ferdinand LA, et al. Providing Patient-Centered Culturally Sensitive Health Care. Couns Psychol 2007;35(5):679–705.
43. Flores G. Devising, implementing, and evaluating interventions to eliminate health care disparities in minority children. Pediatrics 2009;124(Suppl 3):S214–23.
44. Manoleas P. Integrated primary care and behavioral health services for latinos: A blueprint and research agenda. Soc Work Health Care 2008;47(4):438.
45. Hodgkinson S, Godoy L, Beers LS, et al. Improving Mental Health Access for Low-Income Children and Families in the Primary Care Setting. Pediatrics 2017;139:1.

Integrated Behavioral Health Collaborative Practice Embedded Within the Pediatric Residency Continuity Clinic: Incorporating a Multicultural Lens

Sonia Amin, PhD[a],*, Kristine M. Gibson, MD[b], Derrick Bines, PhD[c]

KEYWORDS

- Integrated behavioral health • Interprofessional education
- Interprofessional collaborative practice • Interprofessional curriculum objectives
- Pediatric residency clinic • Psychology and counseling graduate students

KEY POINTS

- The complexity in biopsychosocial concerns among the pediatric population calls for medical providers to strengthen interprofessional relationships with mental health providers.
- The Healthcare Professionals Accreditation Collaborative has called for deliberate interprofessional educational and collaborative practice opportunities.
- Pediatric residency clinics with embedded integrated behavioral health prepare our future health care workforce for interprofessional collaborative practice and increase the likelihood of achieving the quadruple aim.
- Interprofessional collaborative practices help to mitigate health disparities among diverse populations.
- The Interprofessional Education Collaborative competencies provide a framework to identify shared objectives across multiple accrediting bodies.

INTRODUCTION

These past few decades have witnessed an increase in the number of pediatric patients seeking services for complex medical and mental health concerns.[1,2] The interplay of biopsychosocial concerns can make it difficult for any individual discipline of health care professionals to diagnose and manage all the treatment needs with which

[a] University of California-Berkeley, Berkeley, CA, USA; [b] Western Michigan University Homer Stryker M.D. School of Medicine, 1000 Oakland Drive, Kalamazoo, MI 49008, USA; [c] San Francisco State University, San Francisco, CA, USA
* Corresponding author.
E-mail address: sonia.y.amin@wmich.edu

Pediatr Clin N Am 68 (2021) 659–668
https://doi.org/10.1016/j.pcl.2021.02.005
0031-3955/21/© 2021 Elsevier Inc. All rights reserved.

pediatric.theclinics.com

pediatric patients present.[2] Although mental health concerns are prevalent among pediatric populations, 40% to 80% of children and adolescents are not diagnosed nor do they receive the necessary treatment interventions.[1–3]

Effective treatment management of pediatric patients has increasingly required health care providers to have the requisite skill set to work in interprofessional teams and multidisciplinary settings, as well as possess sociocultural awareness to optimize the health of both their pediatric patients and larger communities.[4,5] Uniprofessional curricula pose serious limitations for health care professionals because it limits the interprofessional communication and teamwork required for comprehensive patient care.[5] Siloed models of care may also translate to medical and psychological conditions being misdiagnosed or undiagnosed, because a single health care discipline cannot possess all the intellectual resources needed to manage the full spectrum of patient needs. One strategy to combat this limited educational focus is to develop interprofessional collaborative practices that can be used during student placements, clinical practica, internships, and residency clinics.[4]

The development of integrated behavioral health (IBH) pediatric residency clinics are examples of models that can have immense rewards for patients, parents, and clinicians as well as meet the emerging mental health needs of children and adolescents.[4] IBH pediatric clinics establish a clear nexus between medical and mental health, because they create interprofessional teams that include attending and resident physicians, mental health professionals, and other health care providers.[4,5] These kinds of IBH programs can help to mitigate the number of pediatric patients whose mental health concerns are often left undiagnosed. The collaborative nature of interprofessional collaborative practices can also decrease the stress and burden of a single health care professional to provide all the needed care for a patient as well as aid health care professionals across disciplines to facilitate diagnosis, interventions, and treatment.[6]

HEALTH CARE INEQUITIES AMONG DIVERSE PEDIATRIC PATIENT POPULATIONS

Pediatric patients from racial minority and other intersectional marginalized backgrounds experience the most harm when health care professionals across disciplines do not possess the necessary sociocultural awareness or skill set needed to provide equitable care for their diverse patient populations.[7,8] The current novel coronavirus disease 2019 pandemic has heightened societal awareness of these health care inequities.[9–11] National data illustrate these health care inequities with the increased rates of infection, hospitalizations, and death among African American, Latinx, and Native American populations.[9–11] The disproportionately high number of African American and racial minority communities contracting the novel coronavirus disease 2019 is not limited to social or socioeconomic conditions, but rather demonstrates the lack of access to and adequate early prevention, treatment, and management of preexisting medical conditions.[10]

Historical medical data, patient narratives, and research have shown that neglecting cultural diversity by not adopting culturally sensitive frameworks into patient interaction and treatment intervention models does a great disservice to patient outcomes.[3,11] Implicit bias often results in inadequate treatment and misdiagnosis of patients from racial minority backgrounds, specifically Black and Latinx patients, as well as differential treatment of patients from lower socioeconomic backgrounds.[12] Health care inequities and cultural bias in the provision of health care service delivery to racial minority children and adolescents has impacted quality of care, morbidity, and mortality rates, which makes this an important area to guide interprofessional educational practice.[3]

INTEGRATED BEHAVIORAL HEALTH COLLABORATIVE PRACTICE
Developing a Shared Curriculum

Interprofessional education (IPE) occurs when "students from two or more professions learn about, from and with each other to enable effective collaboration and improve health outcomes."[12] The IBH primary care model that embeds mental health professionals and learners into pediatric continuity care clinics provides the scaffolding with which to develop shared objectives founded on the 4 Interprofessional Education Collaborative competency domains: values and ethics for interprofessional practice, roles and responsibilities, interprofessional communication, and teams and teamwork.[5,12] In addition, training programs using interprofessional collaborative models are uniquely situated to incorporate a multicultural framework within the values and ethics domain and shift away from professional and hierarchical centering. Applying this multicultural framework will further enhance the evaluation and management of pediatric patients seeking care in their medical home.[13]

Careful curriculum planning must take place to ensure that all learner needs are identified and met. The Accreditation Council for Graduate Medical Education, American Board of Pediatrics, Pediatrics Milestone Project, and Entrustable Professional Activities, as well as the competencies required for the American Psychological Association and Council on Social Work Education intersect with the Interprofessional Education Collaborative competencies, creating opportunities for integrated learning objectives in the clinical setting.[14–16] Faculty from all disciplines represented in the clinic will need to determine how learners will be assigned to cases, the process for patient handoffs, and interprofessional faculty staffing.

SHARED VALUES AND ETHICS
Overlapping and Conflicting Ethical Guidelines Across Professions

Establishing shared values and ethics is fundamental to creating a high functioning team. Medical and mental health disciplines have evolved through different traditions of practice, resulting in often overlapping but conflicting ethical guidelines regarding the care and treatment of patients and clients.[17,18] As examples, owing to American Psychological Association's ethical guidelines restricting multiple relationships as it is viewed as impacting the objectivity of care, psychologists will often not conduct therapy with the family members of their colleagues or have dual relationships with clients receiving ongoing treatment from them.[17] In contrast, it might be more common for physicians to consult with a colleague's family member or friend.[18]

Further, without a recognition and discussion of where interprofessional and cultural competency barriers exist and consensus developed around common vocabulary and workflows, these divergent practices can lead to contradictory care plans. Teams should apply a multicultural framework as they evaluate the differences in values and ethical guidelines of each discipline to understand where discrepancies may emerge. Before clinical assignments are made, individuals in social work or psychology graduate programs are trained in the use of multicultural assessment tools, taking into consideration a patient's cultural context and background as part of assessment, diagnosis, and intervention choices.[17] The medical model of etiology and interventions are quite different. Psychology and pediatrics have unique guidelines regarding professional competencies and the depth, breadth, and timing of curriculum programming may emphasize cultural considerations at differential levels of training.[18] For example, many social work and psychology graduate programs tend to have entire courses focused on multicultural competencies as a part of the foundational course work, which is rarely the case in traditional medical education.[19,20]

A multicultural framework involves an assessment of limitations in the understanding the context of our patients and community members, to provide better treatment and care to them. For example, one that is often up for debate is the concept of what constitutes child abuse and what is informed through cultural child rearing practices. Understanding the cultural context of a pediatric patient may help to distinguish whether the patient is experiencing abuse or culturally informed child rearing practices. This context will enable health care professionals to enact appropriate measures in whether or not to report to child protective services, to develop a behavioral plan, and/or how to engage with the patient and family members. Thus, these can be opportunities for shared learning to take place, which will allow both mental health and medical professionals to be on the same page with their conceptualization and in turn treatment decisions for their patients.

Equity in Funding Allocation, Space, and Decision-Making Powers

Another area that requires deliberate conversation before interprofessional teams can successfully manage the care of their shared patients is to determine what equity looks like with respect to the physical space allocation, funding resources, time, and extent of decision-making in patient care, all of which are important considerations for an effective IBH model.[21,22] Funding is a crucial issue that needs to be discussed, especially when there are multiple academic departments, programs, and institutions that are contributing learners.[21] Funding-related decisions should be discussed before the implementation of IBH programs and should include mental health professionals at the decision-making table.[22] Further, the effectiveness of IBH clinics also depends on creating and maintaining equity among medical and behavioral health providers in the allotment of work stations and technology.[21]

Staffing models are also of critical importance, because the understaffing of behavioral health providers creates additional barriers when pediatric patients are unable to receive care within the holistic treatment model. The question that arises during these challenges is which pediatric patients are deemed as essential to receive IBH services, are they those patients who have already been diagnosed with mental health concerns owing to being able to afford therapy services or those who not only have high stigma of mental illnesses but also are unable to afford outside services? Understaffing can also create divisional hierarchy and calls into question the perceived value that each service provides to patients.[4,21]

ROLES AND RESPONSIBILITIES

Patients receive the most equitable and comprehensive care when health care professionals are able to reflect, engage, and adjust their roles based on patient needs. Thus, it is important to focus on provider expertise and skills rather than on the hierarchy of qualifications when addressing patient needs.[5] Hierarchies present among medical and mental health providers can create additional barriers to the provision of high-quality care when the expertise of all team members is not sought, honored, or incorporated into patient care across disciplines.[19] To decrease professional hierarchies and promote a collaborative orientation, scholars advocate for professionals to view their respective disciplines as subgroups within the broader umbrella of health care professions.[23] Understanding and valuing the roles of other providers can contribute to a more welcoming work environment and promote positive patient outcomes.[23] Health care professionals across disciplines should be taught how to engage with diverse professionals, develop collaborative relationships, and be able to identify their own and others' unique and complementary abilities to optimize health and patient care.

IBH programs provide the needed clinical exposure for providers-in-training to develop a sense of their own cognitive and procedural abilities while collaborating with the broader health care team in a patient centered approach. The care of patients with attention deficit hyperactivity disorder (ADHD) provides a useful example of shifting roles in diagnosis and management. Although it may be common for medical providers to prescribe ADHD medications based on patient and parental reports as well as brief assessment tools, residents in training need to recognize when the expertise of a behavioral health professional is warranted in the diagnostic process, especially given the high rates of overdiagnosis and misdiagnosis of ADHD within pediatric populations.[24] Mental health professionals can conduct comprehensive psychological evaluations when there is a question about the diagnostic accuracy of brief assessments or other concerns noted in the history.[25] IBH professionals are also able to manage some of the functional impairments of ADHD through behavioral therapy approaches.[26] Role awareness, in conjunction with good team communication, allows for the team member with the requisite skill set to take the lead at each phase of the patient care process. The collaborative nature of this model of care lends itself to shared curriculum objectives and provides context to deconstruct hierarchies and decrease bias in determining case leadership.[27]

INTERPROFESSIONAL COMMUNICATION

The competency for interprofessional communication is perhaps the core component of a shared curriculum.[5] This competency refers to communication with patients, families, communities, and other professionals in a way that is, clear and responsible and supports a team-based approach to health care. The subcompetencies for interprofessional communication focus on effective communication tools, understandable language that does not include discipline-specific jargon, clarity and respect, timeliness, and a recognition of how power and hierarchies influence communication.[5] The hierarchies that exist among health care professions need to be addressed within these integrated care models. Additionally, learners and providers should consider relationships between the medical field and community members.

In considering a multicultural framework, cross-cultural exchanges, whether across providers or with patients and community members, should be central in learning. Training programs can implement interprofessional courses or activities in which students are able to participate in shared learning and practice effective communication strategies that can be applied to future patient interactions. The use of case examples can be helpful for exploring cross-professional and cross-cultural scenarios that are likely to present when working with patients. Interprofessional communication is a vital tool in sustaining the relationships among team members, patients, families, and community members.

The extant literature describes a long history of discrimination from those within the medical field toward marginalized communities, namely, African Americans. Medical mistrust refers to a lack of confidence in the medical field, including providers, as a response to a history of mistreatment and experiences of discrimination within health care.[28] This mistrust may result in a skepticism in what is being communicated by providers and a hesitance to seek treatment. Health care professionals should seek to mitigate this mistrust by building relationships, listening and attending to community needs, and communicating truthfully and clearly. These considerations can begin to actualize as they are incorporated into training programs. The Society of General

Internal Medicine's Health Equity Commission (formerly the Health Disparities Task Force) offered recommendations for training programs that focus on 3 areas of curricula: examine and understand attitudes that may impact clinical encounters, gain knowledge of health disparities and the solutions to decrease and eliminate them, and acquire skills to effectively communicate across cultures, languages, and literacy levels.[29] The American Psychological Association Multicultural Guidelines offer supplemental guidance for providers and learners to consider their own social identities, those of their peers, and patients, and how these identities may inform their experiences in health care and in the world.[30]

TEAMS AND TEAMWORK

When interprofessional programming is discussed, especially around IBH, institutions need to consider how to create an environment where both medical and mental health providers feel like they are part of a team versus remaining in individual siloes. Understanding one's scope of practice and discerning when to step back or spend more time with the patient is an important skill set to develop when providing interprofessional team-based care.[5] The existent guidelines suggest that learning objectives should focus on having learners practice relationship-fostering values and team dynamics in interprofessional settings.[13] Furthermore, it is important that a core component involves an assessment of multicultural skills in the team environment.

Team members from diverse cultural backgrounds may view teamwork in different ways. Thus, in addition to considering expertise, personalities, approaches, and disciplines, it is important to discuss cultural values and understanding of teamwork, because these differences may manifest via disagreements among team members.[31] For example, expectations and ideas around leadership may differ across cultures, demonstrated through differences in individualistic and collectivistic cultural norms. Additionally, how confident does each health care professional team feel in their awareness and abilities to address racism, sexism, homophobia, and other intersectional variables within the team environment and in turn patient care?[32] Ongoing assessment and training to foster multicultural awareness and competency in the staffing teams is essential in the development of an IBH program, that aims to provide holistic and culturally sensitive care to its patient populations.[32]

Thus, team success also depends on its members' ability to reflect on biases and privileges among individual and team members in rating performances. This practice can be modeled by faculty, who can not only exhibit critical consciousness, but also effective teamwork with faculty across disciplines. Trainees tend to internalize and model the behaviors they observe by those they respect in their fields. Thus, it can also be helpful for learners to have practice simulations of what staffing for different case types and patients, and discern where flexibility and adaptability may be required.

Learning opportunities should allow participants to demonstrate effective adaptation to different team roles to plan, deliver, and assess patient-centered care and interventions that are safe, efficient, effective, and equitable.[13] Effective teamwork involves being able to integrate the knowledge and experiences of each health team member to inform decision-making and treatment interventions for pediatric patients.[5] Teams must also develop a process to review the knowledge base and skill set required to effectively manage patient visits and determine which team members will be involved during the patient encounter. Although patients and families may only meet face to face with a few providers, many health professionals may be working together to provide care. Any discrepancies, conflicts, or contradictory information delivered to the patient may hinder a health care team's ability to provide adequate care to the patient. Therefore, expectations for effective teamwork and managing team dynamics are important to address in interprofessional practices.

BENEFITS OF INTEGRATED BEHAVIORAL HEALTH COLLABORATIVE PRACTICE

Racial and ethnic minority populations have a relatively high stigma toward mental illnesses and, combined with historical inequities, this lack of access to physical and mental health care services contributes to the low use rates of mental health services.[33] An IBH model can mitigate this barrier because it incorporates mental and emotional health into a holistic pediatric patient care team. Having providers work side by side allows for the introduction of mental health services for patients who may not have independent access to these services or possess elevated levels of stigma associated with mental illnesses. Pediatric patients often have mental health concerns that go untreated because families fail to seek out mental health services owing to stigma, a lack of awareness, or a misunderstanding of mental illnesses.[6] Another benefit of an embedded IBH practice is that pediatric patients from lower income backgrounds, who may have limited access to mental health services owing to a lack of insurance coverage or high copayments, are able to access IBH services that are included as part of the medical health care visit.[6] Behavioral health providers are able to spend additional time with the patient, approach them with sociocultural awareness, and establish a sense of trust. This practice can result in the collection of a more in-depth history surrounding the patient's concerns, but may also contradict information gathered by the physician. Providers will then need to use their interprofessional teamwork and communication skills to shape a holistic narrative of the patient and their concerns, review potential etiologies, and develop comprehensive treatment plans.

INTEGRATED BEHAVIORAL HEALTH IMPLEMENTATION AND BARRIERS TO SUCCESS

Institutions must respond to the challenges of interprofessional training by developing unique programs that incorporate multicultural competency and take into consideration the strengths and resources available in their regions.[4,31] Although there are clear benefits to interprofessional collaborative practices, there are also real challenges inherent in developing and facilitating culturally sensitive IPE training events, planning a longitudinal IPE curriculum, and implementing effective interprofessional collaborative practices. The first step for program success requires interprofessional educational partners to work together to develop an overarching and culturally informed IPE curriculum approach.[34] Programs should complete a local needs assessment (eg, patient and community demographics, income levels, funding resources and grants, and center culture), which will allow programs to assess what resources exist and additional needs that will be needed to implement an effective IBH curriculum at their institution.[35] Direct discussions about practice models (fully integrated vs colocated), space for learners and faculty, access to medical records, confidentiality, funding streams, and insurance coverage will all be necessary discussion points to plan for success.

When developing curriculum at the graduate medical, psychological, counseling, and social work levels, individual programs will need to define competency targets for each phase or level of learner.[16] Faculty will then need to pair the correct levels of learners for practice in the collaborative setting, ensuring that the prerequisite skills have been developed before practice in the clinical environment.[18] IPE opportunities before collaborative practice can be provided through case-based and simulated opportunities for teams to practice core skills before application with patients.

The sustainability of the IBH model will require financial planning to determine how reimbursement models based on payer policies affects institutional abilities to develop and administer quality interprofessional curriculum and practices.[4] An assessment of whether IBH appointments are covered individually or folded into the overall well child appointment will inform the level of institutional funding required to support mental health learners and faculty. Discrepancies in billing often create barriers and can hinder effective patient care integration, because it contributes to the hierarchy within the staffing team.[29]

SUMMARY

IBH programs create an effective bridge between mental health and medical disciplines and, in turn, enable health care institutions to provide holistic care to their pediatric patient populations. Further, interprofessional practices that have in its core component, multicultural competency skills, allows for health care professionals across disciplines to not only dismantle hierarchy across disciplines but also contextualize through a cultural lens patient experiences and barriers, which will aid in building rapport, trust, and adherence to treatment interventions.

CLINICS CARE POINTS

- Pediatric patients require an integrated pediatric team to provide adequate care for complex medical and mental health concerns.
- Implicit bias training needs to be implemented in health care institutions to provide culturally sensitive health care services to historically marginalized communities.
- A community assessment can provide valuable information about the demographics and needs of the community, allowing for a better understanding of how to structure integrated care.
- Pediatric health care service delivery models need to incorporate an integrated behavioral model to assess for psychological and behavioral health concerns, which are often underdiagnosed within this population.
- Health care models should embed training and health care staffing models that focus on practicing effective communication, teamwork practices, roles and responsibilities, shared values and ethics, and equitable status in interdisciplinary teams.

DISCLOSURE

The authors have nothing to disclose.

REFERENCES

1. Data and Statistics on Children's Mental Health | CDC. Available at: https://www.cdc.gov/childrensmentalhealth/data.html. Accessed September 13, 2020.
2. Watanabe-Galloway S, Valleley R, Rieke K, et al. Behavioral health problems presented to integrated pediatric behavioral health clinics: differences in urban and rural patients. Community Ment Health J 2017;53(1):27–33.
3. Howell E, McFeeters J. Children's mental health care: differences by race/ethnicity in urban/rural areas. J Health Care Poor Underserved 2008;19:237–47.

4. McMillan JA, Land M, Leslie LK. Pediatric residency education and the behavioral and mental health crisis: a call to action. Pediatrics 2017;139(1). https://doi.org/10.1542/peds.2016-2141.

5. Bachynsky N. Implications for policy: the triple aim, quadruple aim, and interprofessional collaboration. Nurs Forum 2020;55(1):54–64.

6. Education Collaborative Expert Panel I. Sponsored by the interprofessional education collaborative* report of an expert panel core competencies for interprofessional collaborative practice 2011. Available at: https://nebula.wsimg.com/3ee8a4b5b5f7ab794c742b14601d5f23. Accessed August 28, 2020.

7. Williams DR, Rucker TD. Understanding and addressing racial disparities in health care. Health Care Financ Rev 2000;21(4):75–90.

8. Richmond A, Jackson J. Cultural considerations for psychologists in primary care. J Clin Psychol Med Settings 2018;25(3):305–15.

9. Flores G. Technical report-racial and ethnic disparities in the health and health care of children. Pediatrics 2010;125:979.

10. Tai DBG, Shah A, Doubeni CA, et al. The disproportionate impact of COVID-19 on racial and ethnic minorities in the United States. Clin Infect Dis 2020. https://doi.org/10.1093/cid/ciaa815.

11. Chowkwanyun M, Reed AL Jr. Racial health disparities and Covid-19 - caution and context. N Engl J Med 2020. https://doi.org/10.1056/NEJMp2012910.

12. Health Professions Accreditors Collaborative. Guidance on Developing Quality Interprofessional Education for Health Professions; 2019.

13. Todd KH, Lee THJ. The effect of ethnicity on physician estimates of pain severity in patients with isolated extremity trauma. JAMA 1994;271(12):925–8.

14. Gilbert JHV, Yan J, Hoffman SJ. A WHO report: framework for action on interprofessional education and collaborative practice. J Allied Health 2010;39(SUPPL. 1):196–7.

15. ACGME Pediatrics Milestone Project. Available at: https://www.acgme.org/Portals/0/PDFs/Milestones/PediatricsMilestones.pdf. Accessed June 22, 2020.

16. Entrustable Professional Activities for General Pediatrics. Available at: https://www.abp.org/entrustable-professional-activities-epas. Accessed June 22, 2020.

17. American Psychological Association. Standards of accreditation for health service psychology. 2015;(August 2017):1-50.

18. Kaddari MF, Koslowsky M, Weingarten MA. Ethical behaviour of physicians and psychologists: similarities and differences. J Med Ethics 2017;1–4.

19. Freeth D, Hammick M, Reeves S, et al. In: Freeth DS, Hammick M, Scott R, et al, editors. Effective interprofessional education: development, delivery, and evaluation. Blackwell Publishing Ltd; 2005.

20. Boland DH, Juntunen CL, Kim HY, et al. Integrated behavioral health curriculum in counseling psychology training programs. Couns Psychol 2019;47(7):1012–36.

21. Integration of depression and primary care: barriers to adoption. J Prim Care Community Heal 2014. https://doi.org/10.1177/2150131913491290.

22. Kelsay K, Bunik M, Buchholz M, et al. Incorporating trainees' development into a multidisciplinary training model for integrated behavioral health within a pediatric continuity clinic. Child Adolesc Psychiatr Clin N Am 2017;26(4):703–15.

23. McNair RP. The case for educating health care students in professionalism as the core content of interprofessional education. Med Educ 2005;39(5):456–64.

24. Ford-Jones PC. Misdiagnosis of attention deficit hyperactivity disorder: "Normal behaviour" and relative maturity. Paediatr Child Heal 2015;20(4):200–2.

25. Padwa H, Teruya C, Tran E, et al. The implementation of integrated behavioral health protocols in primary care settings in project care. J Subst Abuse Treat 2016;62:74–83.

26. Standards of Accreditation for Programs in Health Service Psychology and Accreditation Operating Procedures. Available at: https://www.apa.org/ed/accreditation/about/policies/standards-of-accreditation.pdf. Accessed June 22, 2020.

27. NASW. Standards and indicators for cultural competence in social work practice. Natl Comm Racial Ethn Divers Natl Comm Racial Ethn Divers. Published online 2015:2014-2016. Available at: https://www.socialworkers.org/LinkClick.aspx?fileticket=7dVckZAYUmk%3D&portalid=0. Accessed September 18, 2020.

28. Howell E. Access to Children's Mental Health Services under Medicaid and SCHIP. 2004;Series B(B-60):1-8. Available at: https://www.mendeley.com/catalogue/31fa7bed-7b36-3024-be67-6f044cf7b534/?utm_source=desktop&utm_medium=1.19.4&utm_campaign=open_catalog&userDocumentId=%7B1951705f-4f96-410e-b6ae-a47441ad1ed9%7D. Accessed September 15, 2020.

29. Smith WR, Betancourt JR, Wynia MK, et al. Recommendations for teaching about racial and ethnic disparities in health and health care. Ann Intern Med 2007; 147(9):654–5.

30. Multicultural guidelines: an ecological approach to context, identity, and intersectionality, 2017 Prepared by the Task Force on Re-Envisioning the Multicultural Guidelines for the 21st Century Adopted by the APA Council of Representatives in August 2017 Overall List of Multicultural Guidelines 4. Available at: http://www.apa.org/about/policy/multicultural-guidelines.pdf. Accessed September 19, 2020.

31. Wolraich ML, Hagan JF, Allan C, et al. Clinical practice guideline for the diagnosis, evaluation, and treatment of attention-deficit/hyperactivity disorder in children and adolescents. Pediatrics 2019;144(4). https://doi.org/10.1542/peds.2019-2528.

32. Hope JM, Lugassy D, Meyer R, et al. Bringing interdisciplinary and multicultural team building to health education: the downstate team-building initiative. Acad Med 2005;80(1):74–83.

33. Harper JC. IPEC's core competency 2 roles and responsibilities: what more do we need to implement these? J Nurs Educ Pract 2019;9(7):46.

34. Parker K, Jacobson A, McGuire M, et al. How to build high-quality interprofessional collaboration and education in your hospital: the IP-COMPASS tool. Qual Manag Health Care 2012;21(3):160–8.

35. Ball K, Lawson W, Alim T. Medical mistrust, conspiracy beliefs & HIV-related behavior among African Americans. J Psychol Behav Sci 2013;1(1):1–7. Available at: http://aripd.org/journals/jpbs/Vol_1_No_1_December_2013/1.pdf.

Integrated Behavioral Health and Intervention Models

Mark S. Barajas, PhD[a],*, Derrick Bines, PhD[b],
Jason Straussman, MSW[c]

KEYWORDS

- IBH models • Interventions • Biopsychosocial model • Motivational interviewing

KEY POINTS

- Integrating physical and mental health care is a national priority.
- The National Institute on Mental Health endorses 3 integrated behavioral health models.
- Mental health accounts for approximately 25% of worldwide illness.
- Social workers and psychologists are well-positioned to contribute to integrated behavioral health.

As evidence has grown documenting the connection between physical and emotional well-being, greater interest and resources have been devoted to developing holistic systems of health care.[1] One key piece of data emerging from decades of research is the high percentage of patients for whom primary care was the first place they discussed mental or emotional concerns.[2] Thus, recognizing the need for a better integration of physical and emotional health care, several branches of allied health began conceptualizing models of training for the next generation of health care workers.

This article explores models of integrated behavioral health (IBH) with a focus on the principles, training, and experiences of social workers and psychologists working in IBH settings. First, a conceptual framework for understanding integrated care is discussed and an overview of 3 models will be presented. Next, we focus on the unique contributions of 2 mental health disciplines, namely, social work and psychology, and particular interventions well-suited for use in IBH settings. Finally, we share information about specific training requirements and the experiences of social workers and psychologists working in IBH settings.

[a] Department of Psychology, Saint Mary's College of California, 1928 St Mary's Road, Moraga, CA 94575, USA; [b] Department of Counseling, San Francisco State University, 1600 Holloway Avenue, Burk Hall, Room 524, San Francisco, CA 94132, USA; [c] Tang Counseling Center, University of California, 2222 Bancroft Way, Berkeley, CA 94720, USA
* Corresponding author.
E-mail address: mb37@stmarys-ca.edu

Pediatr Clin N Am 68 (2021) 669–683
https://doi.org/10.1016/j.pcl.2021.02.015
0031-3955/21/© 2021 Elsevier Inc. All rights reserved.

INTEGRATED BEHAVIORAL HEALTH MODELS

IBH care models, also referred to as integrated care models, combine primary care and behavioral health care services in a single setting. Developed as a conceptual framework by the National Council for Community Behavioral Healthcare, the 4 quadrant clinical integration model describes the degree of integration for particular settings and which settings are best suited to provide patient care, based on the severity of presenting concerns.[3] An overview of the model is provided in **Table 1**.

Although the 4 quadrant clinical integration model provides an understanding of the types of settings that are best suited for particular populations, specific IBH models provide insight to how care is provided in a particular setting. The National Institute on Mental Health describes 3 IBH models, namely, collaborative care, patient-centered medical homes (PCMH), and hub-based systems.[4] We provide an overview of these IBH models and review the strengths and limitations of each.

Collaborative Care

Collaborative care is a team-based treatment approach that incorporates behavioral health care and consultations with mental health specialists into primary care.[4] The collaborative team is often composed of a primary care provider, care management staff (eg, nurse, social worker, or psychologist), and a psychiatric consultant.[5] The primary care provider monitors patient symptoms and adjusts treatment systematically according to patient needs, requests, and progress. The care management staff may provide brief behavioral interventions or brief psychotherapy, such as cognitive behavioral therapy, and consults regularly with the psychiatrist about treatment planning.[5] The psychiatric consultant advises about patients whose symptoms do not improve. Patients who require a higher level of care may be referred to mental health specialty care.[5]

The current literature highlights the benefits and challenges of using a collaborative care approach to treatment. Adult patients treated using a collaborative care model have experienced sustained decrease in anxiety and depression symptoms up to 2 years after their initial treatment.[6,7] These results have been found in mostly White and in ethnic minority samples. Additionally, patients treated within a collaborative care model have shown greater adherence to medication use guidance, improved quality of life, and greater satisfaction with treatment.[6] Adolescents treated within a

Table 1		
Four quadrant clinical integration model (brief description)		
Quadrant	**Description**	
Quadrant 1	*Concerns*: Low behavioral health and low physical health care needs. *Setting*: Primary care setting with behavioral health care staff on site.	
Quadrant 2	*Concerns*: High behavioral health and physical health care needs. *Setting*: Behavioral health care setting that coordinates with a primary care provider.	
Quadrant 3	*Concerns*: Low behavioral health and high physical health care needs. *Setting*: Primary care setting with behavioral health care staff in primary care.	
Quadrant 4	*Concerns*: High behavioral health and high physical health care needs. *Setting*: Fully integrated setting that can offer mental health and substance use care.	

Note. Adopted from Mauer et al., 2005.

collaborative care model have exhibited less severe behavior problems and lower levels of hyperactivity, anxiety, and depression compared with those treated in a nonintegrated model.[8] Challenges to collaborative care include those that are clinical (eg, provider difficulty with distinguishing physical and mood symptoms and patient–provider communication), organizational (eg, access to care and limited time for mental health evaluations), and financial (eg, reimbursement for mental health treatment).[9] One case study that examined the implementation of a collaborative care model in a community-based setting serving primarily low-income, Latinx patients found that barriers to implementation included the lack of a thorough understanding of clinic systems and processes, limited resources, and relationships among collaborative care team members.[10]

Patient-Centered Medical Home

A PCMH is an integrated care model in which patients have access to a provider who coordinates their care to ensure that their needs are met and that treatment goals are communicated clearly.[4] The American Academy of Family Physicians, American Academy of Pediatrics, American College of Physicians, and the American Osteopathic Association founded the joint principles to describe the ideal characteristics of PCMH. These principles include:

1. A personal physician who maintains an ongoing relationship with each patient;
2. The personal physician leads a team that provides care for each patient;
3. The personal physician is responsible for all the patient's health care needs, or arranges the appropriate supports;
4. Care is coordinated across elements of the health care system and provides patients with social and medical resources;
5. Attention to quality and safety;
6. Enhanced access to care; and
7. A payment structure that values the work of the personal physician and other staff members.[11]

Baird and colleagues[12] offered a supplemental set of behavioral joint principles to emphasize the centrality of behavioral health care into the PCMH model. They described factors necessary to achieve these principles, such as improvements for collaboration among providers, training, research, and the inclusion of behavioral health services on benefit plans.

A review of the current literature reveals the advantages and challenges related to the PCMH model. Among the advantages, PCMHs offer increased access to care, more engagement with providers, and improved quality of care.[13] Additionally, the PCMH model offers financial benefits that are achieved through fewer inpatient and emergency department visits, and decreased hospital readmission rates.[14] Alternatively, the limitations of PCMH models include inconclusive patient results and insufficient evidence of sustained outcomes, potential financial losses for independent practices, challenges with coordinating care among providers, and the length of time necessary to implement the model into a health care system.[13,15,16]

Hub-Based Systems

The third IBH care model outlined by National Institute on Mental Health is the hub-based approach. This system follows the model of the Massachusetts Child Psychiatry Access Project, which allows for direct consultation with a child psychiatrist via telephone, immediate in-person clinical consultation, and care coordination.[4] The Massachusetts Child Psychiatry Access Project is a statewide system consisting of regional child behavioral health consultation hubs that include a child psychiatrist, a licensed therapist, and a care coordinator.[17] Noted strengths of hub-based models are their accessibility, their individualized approach to supporting primary care providers, and their specific focus on pediatric providers.[17] A challenge of this model is that care is focused within primary care settings. Although care coordinators can facilitate access to resources outside of what is provided within the primary care, insurance policies may not cover such outside support or the outside resources may have a limited capacity to be supportive. Other limitations include the differing availability of resources based on region and, unlike other integrated models (eg, PMCH), mental health professionals are off site, which can be a barrier for supporting patients.[17]

Integrated health care models ultimately seek to decrease barriers to patient care by combining care services in a way that increases accessibility. Key differences among the collaborative care, PCMH, and hub-based models include the location of service providers (ie, in a single setting or remote) and the emphasis on patient-centered care compared with provider-centered support. Given their focus on patient-centered care and collaboration, mental health professionals provide a unique contribution to health care. These contributions are discussed elsewhere in this article.

THE IMPORTANCE OF MENTAL HEALTH

Global health care reform has helped to reveal the importance of mental health to a person's overall well-being.[18] According to conclusions reached by recent meta-analyses of health care use, mental health accounts for 25% of all illnesses worldwide.[19,20] Globally, the World Health Organization continues to advocate for greater access to mental health services,[19] and in the United States, public health policy (eg, the Affordable Care Act) has been central in the last 2 presidential campaigns.[21] Health care professionals improve access for marginalized communities by destigmatizing mental health and integrating care.[22] Health care systems are responding to the need for more robust mental health services through new models of care delivery and interdisciplinary collaboration with mental health professions such as social work and counseling psychology.

Social workers and counseling psychologists contribute necessary skills as frontline workers and bring culturally relevant frameworks to meet the diverse needs of clients who seek health services. Social workers in primary care settings increase mental health access and equity through collaborative care and a social justice framework.[23] Counseling psychologists also advance integration through core values of the field[18] and adapt treatment models for brief interventions in health care settings.

Social Work

Social work is an interdisciplinary profession with deep roots in social justice and advocacy. The National Center for Interprofessional Practice and Education proposes that social workers take a leading role in IBH owing to the strong interdisciplinary nature of the field.[23] Social work provides the biopsychosocial model and person-centered care[24] as 2 frameworks for integration.

Biopsychosocial model

George Engel[25] developed the biopsychosocial model as a framework for assessing the biological, psychological, and social impacts on health.[26] The biopsychosocial model calls attention to the ways in which culture, family, nutrition, and community affect patient outcomes.[27] Over time, the biopsychosocial model has been extended to include spirituality, sexuality, and other dimensions of intersectionality, attempting to encompass the unique needs of LGBTQ+ folks and queer women of color.[28,29]

The biopsychosocial model highlights the interplay between mind and body and can inform all levels of patient interaction.[30] Studies on holistic health and healing[31] confirm how social support, culture, health, diet, and spirituality promote wellness. Moreover, findings from studies with refugee populations highlight the phenomenological nature of distress (known as *idioms of distress*) and the importance of language when working cross-culturally.

For example, within the Karen community, a cultural group originally from the Himalayas, participants who had been displaced to Australia described their symptoms as "no one holding their heart" rather than feeling "depressed."[31–35] The biopsychosocial model is particularly useful when working with complex cases because it reminds clinicians to consider patients' language, culture, and family.[36] Although the biopsychosocial model is already integrated in some health care settings, we believe it will gain more prominence as the need for holistic care continues to be recognized worldwide.[26]

Person-centered care

Person-centered care is a driving principle behind global health care reforms and emphasizes collaboration, unconditional positive regard, and empathy.[37,38] Person-centered care shifts medical care away from a top–down approach organized by differential diagnosis[30] and encourages the development of individually tailored treatment plans via patient–clinician collaboration.[39] By treating patients as experts of their own experience,[40] patients become collaborators and cohealers in the process of recovery and illness management.[41] Patients receiving care within a person-centered care model report greater satisfaction, higher rates of recovery, and spending less on health care costs.[41] Person-centered care has also been shown to improve access for marginalized communities[42] and to decrease health inequalities.[43] To better serve under-represented communities, health care workers can learn from person-centered care's model of partnering with patients.

Counseling Psychology

Counseling psychology evolves out of the field of psychology to provide culturally relevant and patient centered care in a wide variety of clinical settings. Counseling psychologists lead in integrative settings as behavioral health specialists through training in interprofessional treatment, cultural humility, and patient centered treatment. Counseling psychologists are guided by a set of core values that contribute to the mission of increasing patient centered and contextual care in health care settings.[21] Core values of counseling psychologists include growth toward the patient's full potential, holistic and contextual care, diversity and social justice, and a communitarian perspective.[44]

Core values

Counseling psychologists strengthen integrative settings through core values of the profession and clinical skills of generalist intervention, rapport building, cultural humility,[45] case management, and coordinated care.[46] These skills increase person-centered care and can be used by other health care workers at various levels of patient interaction. For example, counseling psychologist's commitment to growth toward patients' full potential expands the dichotomy of sick versus healthy to encompass well-being, happiness, and fulfillment.[47] Recidivism and high patient drop-out rates are chronic issues in health care treatment that create financial burdens for health systems. Focusing on patient growth shifts the framework of medicine from symptom reduction to human flourishing and healing. Counseling psychologists sustain growth by eliciting a patient's own understanding of wellness and setting goals based on long-term health.[44] For this reason, the values of fulfillment and contextual care add to the field of medicine and the global mandate for patient centered care.[46] Contextual care and holistic interventions incorporate patient feedback and can guide health care settings to treat the whole patient. Contextual care amplifies patient-centered care and uses holistic interventions such as movement, spiritual practices, acupuncture, and massage[48] to meet the specific needs of patients. Every patient is unique and healing is a personal and phenomenological journey.[49] Similar to the biopsychosocial model, the framework of contextual care provides targeted and patient driven treatment that would benefit integrative settings.

The third and fourth values of social justice and the communitarian perspective[50] address health disparities within marginalized communities. Settings with counseling psychologists have reported better outcomes for marginalized communities and less stigma related to seeking mental health services.[42] Many of these health inequalities are due to lack of access and coordinated care.[45] In addition, the stigma assigned to mental health means that integrative settings can help unlock barriers to treatment. One counseling psychologists working in a primary care setting notes, "we are receiving patients who would never walk through the door."[46] In addition to stigma, systemic racism and implicit bias are major factors in health disparities and health conditions in marginalized communities.[51] Racism and social inequality affect mental and physical health and must be addressed to improve health care treatment for diverse populations. Counseling psychologists challenge systemic oppression through advocacy for clients and drawing on the strengths of the community.[47] A social justice framework advances care for marginalized communities and works to destigmatize mental health.

Evidence-Based Practices

Motivational interviewing

Motivational interviewing increases patient compliance and health through therapeutic and communicative interventions designed to elicit change.[52] A recent meta-analysis of motivational interviewing confirmed treatment efficacy for a range of presenting concerns, including HIV medication compliance, dental hygiene, body weight, alcohol and tobacco use, sedentary behavior, self-monitoring, and confidence in change.[53] Cross-cultural studies in Hong Kong substantiate similar outcomes and suggest that motivational interviewing is useful in a variety of cultural contexts.[54] Motivational interviewing has also been shown to increase patient satisfaction with treatment and decreases recidivism.[54] Motivational interviewing facilitates collaborative healing by eliciting change and moving with resistance. Although brief, motivational interviewing builds trust and rapport, making treatment more direct and effective. Motivational interviewing should be considered at all levels of patient care and saves time and resources for health care professionals, balancing shareholder demands and large caseloads.

Mindfulness-based interventions

Mindfulness-based stress reduction is an evidenced-based model combining Buddhist practice and Western psychology, and seeks to alleviate symptoms via meditation and self-compassion.[55] Studies on mindfulness-based stress reduction reveal decreases in symptoms of depression and anxiety,[56] and increases in general well-being.[57,58] Although mindfulness-based stress reduction was initially designed to treat chronic pain and associated conditions[59] and is easily incorporated into chronic pain clinics and programs, it has also been incorporated into primary care. Similarly, even though mindfulness-based stress reduction was originally designed as a group therapy intervention, mindfulness-based interventions are being incorporated into a wide range of institutions, including schools, work, athletics, nonprofits, and politics.[59] Moreover, mindfulness interventions are easy to implement through phone apps, patient portals, and outpatient groups, making them flexible and cost effective.

Summary

Mental health continues to be recognized as a central issue within health systems. The biopsychosocial model, person-centered care, and the 4 core values of counseling psychology provide holistic frameworks to support this transition. In addition, motivational interviewing and mindfulness-based interventions are evidenced based practices that can be integrated into different levels of patient care. To better understand how counseling psychologists and social workers contribute to integrative models, we now turn to a description of the training both undergo and provide examples from the field. This section explores how training practices and professional standards for both social workers and psychologists are being adapted to serve IBH models.

TRAINING AND EXPERIENCES
General Clinical Training

Although a thorough review of training and licensure requirements for social workers and psychologists is beyond the scope of this article, a brief overview is warranted. It should also be noted that, although variations of social work and psychology graduate programs exist, this section focuses exclusively on programs leading to professional licensure as either a social worker or a psychologist.

In general, licensure as a social worker requires a master's degree and 1 to 2 years of supervised practice. The typical social work curriculum spans 2 years and covers both general (eg, human development, counseling theories) and specialized (eg, psychopathology, school-based interventions) topics, depending on the program's specific focus. Additionally, the social work curriculum contains courses highlighting the impact of sociopolitical systems on individuals (eg, health policy, drug policy) and courses exploring the broad intersection of culture and mental health (eg, social work with immigrants; social work with incarcerated people). Concurrent with theoretic coursework are field-based practicum experiences, where social work students learn and practice clinical skills; sometimes first with each other via role playing and then later with actual clients. After the completion of the master's degree, social work students must then complete approximately 3000 hours (actual number varies slightly by state) of supervised clinical experience and pass a national licensing examination.[60]

The requirements for licensure as a psychologist are similar to those for social work, with only a few differences. First, licensure as a psychologist requires a doctoral degree with coursework typically lasting 3 to 4 years. Supplementing the general and specialized coursework found in social work curricula, doctoral education in counseling and clinical psychology also contains coursework examining the biological aspects of behavior, the diagnosis and treatment of severe mental illness, research design and statistics, and psychological assessment. Similar to social work, doctoral psychology programs also require coursework exploring the intersection of culture and mental health and, depending on the program's focus, may require additional

specialized coursework (eg, clinical supervision, professional consultation) in a particular area. After completion of the doctoral degree, psychology students must then
complete approximately 4000 hours (actual number varies slightly by state) of supervised clinical experience and pass a national licensing examination.[61]

As noted elsewhere in this article, social workers and psychologists share similar
educational trajectories and hold in common a dedication to culturally relevant care
and an awareness of the ways in which systems of care disproportionally confer advantages and disadvantages depending on particular patient demographics (eg,
ethnicity, socioeconomic status), contributing to widespread health disparities.[62]
One attempt at addressing health disparities has been through the conceptualization
and implementation of IBH models.

Integrated Behavioral Health Educational Standards

Although the idea of integrated care is not new, it has received greater attention and
funding over the past 2 decades, partially owing to federal government programs (ie,
2001's New Freedom Commission on Mental Health; 2010's Patient Protection and
Affordable Care Act) specifically emphasizing the need for health care, which addresses both the physical and emotional needs of patients. In 2009, as a part of this
renewed interest, 6 national associations of schools of health professions (eg, American Association of Colleges of Nursing) established the Interprofessional Education
Collaborative (IEPC) and later published the first *Core Competencies for Interprofessional Collaborative Practice*,[63] referred to hereafter as the core competencies. Immediately after publishing the core competencies, 12 additional professional health
organizations, including the Council on Social Work Education and the American Psychological Association, joined the IEPC and helped to publish revised core competencies in 2016[64]; currently, the IEPC provides guidance to more than 60 allied
health professions (eg, dentistry, optometry, and radiology).

IEPC's core competencies are divided into 4 domains (ie, values and ethics; roles
and responsibilities, teams and teamwork, and interprofessional communication)
and are intended to shape the training of students from various health professions
so that they are well prepared to work efficiently in interdisciplinary teams.[63] The
core competencies are guided by shared principles (eg, patient-centered care) and
further operationalized via subcompetencies (eg, develop a trusting relationship with
patients, families, and other team members). Since 2014, both the American Psychological Association and the National Association of Social Workers have developed
more detailed, profession-specific guidelines supplementing the original core
competencies.[24,65]

For psychologists, guidelines for working in integrated health care settings were
published in 2014[65] and are based off work that began as a 2012 American Psychological Association Presidential Initiative. The guidelines, officially named the *Competencies for Psychology Practice in Primary Care* and hereafter referred to as the
primary care competencies, are divided into 6 clusters, each with associated competencies (**Table 2**). To further guide the implementation and evaluation of the primary
care competencies, each competency group is further broken down into essential
components that are operationalized by sample behaviors. For example, "conducts
an evidence-based suicide assessment on all patients identified with depressed
mood" is offered as a sample behavior for the essential component of "assesses pertinent behavioral risk factors" within the assessment competency group of the application cluster.[65]

For social workers, revised guidelines for working in integrated health care settings
were published in 2016 by the National Association of Social Workers and are derived

Table 2
Primary care psychology clusters and competencies

Cluster	Competency Groups
Science	Biopsychosocial approach Research and evaluation
Systems	Leadership and administration Interdisciplinary systems Advocacy
Professionalism	Values and attitudes Diversity Ethics Reflective practice
Relationships	Interprofessionalism Making and maintaining
Application	Practice management Assessment Intervention Clinical consultation
Education	Teaching Supervision

from standards first developed in 2005. The standards, officially known as the *NASW Standards for Social Work Practice in Health Care Settings*, and hereafter referred to as the NASW standards, are grounded by 6 guiding principles of social work (eg, strength-based approach) and further broken down into 13 discrete areas (**Table 3**). Similar to psychology's primary care competencies, the NASW standards are operationalized by example behaviors. For example, "adhere to supervision requirements" is given as a sample behavior under the "qualifications" standard.[24]

Integrated Behavioral Health Training Programs

Building off the theoretic frameworks discussed elsewhere in this article and reflecting the growing awareness that training deficiencies of mental health clinicians are holding back integrated behavioral care efforts,[66] some social work and psychology graduate

Table 3
Principles and standards for social workers in health care

Guiding Principles	Standards
Self-determination	Ethics and values Qualifications
Cultural competency	Knowledge Cultural and linguistic competence
Person-in-environment framework	Screening and assessment Care planning and intervention
Strengths perspective	Advocacy Interdisciplinary collaboration
Primacy of therapeutic relationship	Record keeping and confidentiality Evaluation and quality improvement
Social justice	Workload sustainability Professional development
Importance of research	Supervision and leadership

training programs have begun offering specialized IBH-focused curriculum. For example, The Ohio State University College of Social Work has been developing, with federal financial assistance and in partnership with local community organizations, a training program designed to prepare social workers to "provide community-based IBH care to persons living in underserved communities."[67] Their program, named Integrated and Culturally Relevant Care, is a competitive specialization offered within Ohio State University's general social work curriculum and for which students receive a modest stipend. The Integrated and Culturally Relevant Care is structured around 8 primary learning domains: (1) integrated care, (2) technology in a health care environment, (3) assessment and diagnosis, (4) care coordination and intervention planning, (5) diversity, (6) documentation, (7) health care basics, and (8) evidence-informed behavioral health interventions, and includes robust supervision and frequent student assessment.[67]

Another example is found at New Mexico State University, where, again with federal assistance and local partnerships, all future psychologists are trained under an IBH model that is grounded by psychology's primary care competencies. New Mexico State University's curriculum is structured such that psychology students receive both classroom-based exposure to IBH theory and field-based experiences where they work side by side with other allied health professionals in training (eg, future nurses, pharmacists). Similar to Ohio State University's curriculum, New Mexico State University also provides intensive supervision and ongoing assessment of student skills and knowledge.[68]

Integrated Behavioral Health Experiences

As social work and psychology training programs have evolved to reflect IBH standards, scholars have begun investigating the experiences of licensed clinicians working in IBH settings. Recent studies examining the experiences of social workers in IBH highlight the central role of collaboration and identify 6 frequently used skills[1]: using cultural competency,[2] navigating electronic health records,[3] exploring and responding to patient's social determinants of health,[4] collaborating with other team members,[5] providing patient education,[6] and facilitating communication among team members.[68] Studies also call attention to the feelings of isolation, role confusion, and the systemic priority given to physical health interventions as challenges for social workers working in IBH settings.[69]

Psychologists working in IBH settings have reported similar experiences to their social work colleagues. In addition to individual and group therapy, supervision, and assessment, psychologists working in IBH settings emphasized assertiveness, flexibility, and use of brief interventions as necessary skills.[45] Psychologists also report patient psychoeducation and providing culturally relevant care as key aspects of their professional roles. Regarding challenges, time constraints, emotional exhaustion, and role confusion were among the most common cited by psychologists working in IBH.[45]

SUMMARY

IBH care combines primary and behavioral health care into a common setting. Among the different IBH models, mental health professionals may be colocated with primary care providers in a particular setting, or may be externally located and serve as behavioral health consultants. Regardless of the IBH model, mental health professionals serve as an integral part of the care team. Mental health professionals, namely, social workers and psychologists, contribute a perspective that is informed by extensive theoretic and clinical training. Social workers and psychologists often use treatment models that are strength based, patient centered, consider factors that influence patient experiences (eg, systemic oppression), and that can be incorporated into brief exchanges.

Although contributions are great, mental health professionals may not feel integrated within medical settings. As highlighted elsewhere in this article, mental health professionals may find that their primary care colleagues do not fully understand their role and contribution to the care team. Recent literature suggests that interprofessional training curricula may be helpful in decreasing this confusion. Boland and colleagues[47] provide examples of integrated training curriculums aimed at dispelling stereotypes about behavioral health and medical fields, and educate trainees about the responsibilities of the respective professions. These training models can be helpful in addressing challenges that mental health professionals experience in IBH settings.

CLINICS CARE POINTS

- Treatment delivered within a collaborative care model has been shown to significantly reduce symptoms of anxiety and depression for both White and ethnic minority adults.

- Motivational interviewing and mindfulness-based stress reduction are associated with increases in patient compliance and satisfaction with treatment.

- Future clinicians desiring to work in integrated health care settings are strongly encouraged to seek training opportunities where they can learn along other allied health professionals.

- Clinicians currently working in integrated health care settings are strongly encouraged to clearly articulate roles and responsibilities and regularly discuss scope of practice concerns.

DISCLOSURE

The authors have nothing to disclose.

REFERENCES

1. McDaniel SH, DeGruy FV III. An introduction to primary care psychology. Am Psychol 2014;69(4):325–31.
2. Cherry D, Albert M, McCaig LF. Mental health-related physician office visits by adults aged 18 and over: United States, 2012-2014. NCHS Data Brief, no 311. Hyattville (MD): National Center for Health Statistics; 2018.
3. Mauer B. Integrating behavioral health and primary care services: opportunities and challenges for state mental health authorities. Washington, DC: National Association of State Mental Health Program Directors (NASMHPD) Medical Directors Council; 2005. p. 53. Report No.: 11.
4. National Institute of Mental Health. Integrated care. 2017. Available at: https://www.nimh.nih.gov/health/topics/integrated-care/index.shtml. Accessed May 2, 2020.
5. Unützer J, Henry H, Schoenbaum M, et al. The collaborative care model: an approach for integrating physical and mental health care in Medicaid health homes. Hamilton, New Jersey: Center for Health Care Strategies and Mathematica Policy Research; 2013.
6. Archer J, Bower P, Gilbody S, et al. Collaborative care for depression and anxiety problems. Cochrane Database Syst Rev 2012;10:CD006525.

7. Hu J, Wu T, Damodaran S, et al. The effectiveness of collaborative care on depression outcomes for racial/ethnic minority populations in primary care: a systematic review. Psychosomatics 2020;61(6):632–44.
8. Kolko DJ, Campo J, Kilbourne AM, et al. Collaborative care outcomes for pediatric behavioral health problems: a cluster randomized trial. Pediatrics 2014;133(4): e981–92.
9. Sanchez K. Collaborative care in real-world settings: barriers and opportunities for sustainability. Patient Prefer Adherence 2017;11:71–4.
10. Eghaneyan BH, Sanchez K, Mitschke DB. Implementation of a collaborative care model for the treatment of depression and anxiety in a community health center: results from a qualitative case study. J Multidiscip Healthc 2014;7:503–13.
11. American Academy of Family Physicians, American Academy of Pediatrics, American College of Physicians, American Osteopathic Association. Joint principles of the patient-centered medical home. 2007. Available at: https://www.aafp.org/ dam/AAFP/documents/practice_management/pcmh/initiatives/PCMHJoint.pdf. Accessed May 2, 2020.
12. Working Party Group on Integrated Behavioral Healthcare, Baird M, Blount A, Brungardt S, et al. Joint principles: integrating behavioral health care into the patient-centered medical home. Ann Fam Med 2014;12(2):183–5.
13. Budgen J, Cantiello J. Advantages and disadvantages of the patient-centered medical home: a critical analysis and lessons learned. Health Care Manag (Frederick) 2017;36(4):357–63.
14. Nielsen M, Langner B, Zema C, et al. Benefits of implementing the primary care Patient-centered medical home: a review of cost and quality results. Report from the Patient-Centered Primary Care Collaborative, Washington DC, 2012. p. 1-44
15. Pape SB, Muir S. Primary care occupational therapy: how can we get there? remaining challenges in patient-centered medical homes. Am J Occup Ther 2019; 73(5). 7305090010p1-7305090010p6.
16. Sinaiko AD, Landrum MB, Meyers DJ, et al. Synthesis Of Research On Patient-Centered Medical Homes Brings Systematic Differences Into Relief. Health Aff (Millwood) 2017;36(3):500–8.
17. Straus JH, Sarvet B. Behavioral health care for children: the Massachusetts Child Psychiatry Access Project. Health Aff (Millwood) 2014;33(12):2153–61.
18. Nilsson JE, Berkel LA, Chong WW. Integrated health care and counseling psychology: an introduction to the major contribution. Couns Psychol 2019;47(7): 999–1011.
19. Kroenke K, Unutzer J. Closing the false divide: sustainable approaches to integrating mental health services into primary care. J Gen Intern Med 2017;32(4): 404–10.
20. McAndrew LM, Friedlander ML, Litke DR, et al. Medically unexplained physical symptoms: why counseling psychologists should care about them. Couns Psychol 2019;47(5):741.
21. Golden RL, Vail MR. The implications of the Affordable Care Act for mental health care. Generations 2014;38(3):96–103.
22. Maragakis A, Marianthi N. Hatzigeorgiou. The Transformation of the healthcare system: integrated primary care and the role of Stepped care interventions for behavioral health providers. Principle-based Stepped care and brief psychotherapy for integrated care settings. Cham, Switzerland: Springer International Publishing; 2018.
23. Brandt BF. Memo to social work: it's about the collaboration and the redesign. 2016. National Center for Interprofessional Practice and Education. Available at: https://

nexusipe-resource-exchange.s3.amazonaws.com/CSWE%2011.3.16%20Brandt %20Memo%20to%20Social%20Work.pdf. Accessed June 17, 2020.

24. National Association of Social Workers. NASW standards for social work practice in health care settings. 2016. Available at: https://www.socialworkers.org/ LinkClick.aspx?fileticket=fFnsRHX-4HE%3D&portalid=0. Accessed June 17, 2020.

25. Engel GL. The need for a new medical model: a challenge for biomedicine. Science 1977;196:129–36.

26. Wade DT, Halligan PW. The biopsychosocial model of illness: a model whose time has come. Clin Rehabil 2017;31(8):995–1004.

27. Fisher M, Baum F. The social determinants of mental health: implications for research and health promotion. Aust N Z J Psychiatry 2010;44:1057–63.

28. Henningsen P. Still modern? Developing the biopsychosocial model for the 21st century. J Psychosom Res 2015;79:362–3.

29. Lewis JA, Williams MG, Peppers EJ, et al. Applying Intersectionality to Explore the Relations Between Gendered Racism and Health Among Black Women. J Couns Psychol 2017;64(5):475–86.

30. Stanhope V, Straussner SLA. Social work and integrated health Care: from policy to practice and back. New York: Oxford University Press; 2018.

31. Lane RD. Is it possible to bridge the biopsychosocial model and biomedical models? Biopsychosoc Med 2014;8:3.

32. Niner S, Kokanovic R, Cuthbert D, et al. "Here nobody holds your heart": metaphoric and embodied emotions of birth and displacement among Karen women in Australia. Med Anthropol Q 2014;28(3):362–80.

33. Kleinman A, Benson P. Anthropology in the clinic: the problem of cultural competency and how to fix it. PloS Medicine. 2006. Available at: https://journals.plos. org/plosmedicine/article?id=10.1371/journal.pmed.0030294. Accessed June 20, 2020.

34. Hollifield M, Warner T, Lian N, et al. Measuring trauma and health status in refugees: a critical review. JAMA 2002;288:611–21.

35. Shannon P, O'Dougherty M, Mehta E. Refugees' perspectives on barriers to communication about trauma histories in primary care. Ment Health Fam Med 2012;9(1):47–55.

36. Byrow Y, Pajak R, Specker P, et al. Perceptions of mental health and perceived barriers to mental health help-seeking amongst refugees: a systematic review. Clin Psychol Rev 2020;75:101812.

37. National Institute of Mental Health. Integrated care. Bethesda, MD; 2017. Available at: https://www.nimh.nih.gov/health/topics/integrated-care/index.shtml. Accessed June 17, 2020.

38. Rogers C. On becoming a person: a therapist's view of psychotherapy. London: Constable; 1967.

39. Coulter A, Entwistle VA, Eccles A, et al. Personalised care planning for adults with chronic or long-term health conditions. Cochrane Libr 2015;3.

40. Vreeland B. Bridging the gap between mental and physical health: a multidisciplinary approach. J Clin Psychiatry 2007;68(4):26–33.

41. Rapp CA, Goscha RJ. The strengths model: case management with people with psychiatric disabilities. New York: Oxford University Press; 2006.

42. Kohrt BA, Turner EL, Rai S, et al. Reducing mental illness stigma in healthcare settings: proof of concept for a social contact intervention to address what matters most for primary care providers. Soc Sci Med 2020;250:112852.

43. World Health Organization. Social determinants of health. Geneva (Switzerland): World Health Organization; 2015.

44. Bagayogo IP, Turcios-Wiswe K, Taku K, et al. Providing mental health services in the primary care setting: the experiences and perceptions of general practitioners at a New York City Clinic. Psychiatr Q 2018;89(4):897–908.

45. Berkel LA, Nilsson JE, Joiner AV, et al. Experiences of early career psychologists working in integrated health care. Couns Psychol 2019;47(7):1037–60.

46. Perrin PB, Elliott TR. Setting our sails: counseling psychology in the age of integrated health care. Couns Psychol 2019;47(7):1061–7.

47. Boland DH, Juntunen CL, Kim HY, et al. Integrated behavioral health curriculum in counseling psychology training programs. Couns Psychol 2019;47(7):1012–36.

48. Van der Kolk B. The body keeps the score: brain, mind, and body in the healing of trauma. New York: Penguin Books; 2015.

49. Scott JG, Warber SL, Dieppe P, et al. Healing journey: a qualitative analysis of the healing experiences of Americans suffering from trauma and illness. BMJ open 2017;7(8):e016771.

50. Scheel MJ, Stabb SD, Cohn TJ, et al. Counseling Psychology Model Training Program ψ. Couns Psychol 2018 Jan;46(1):6.

51. Leary JD. Post traumatic slave syndrome: America's legacy of enduring injury and healing. Portland, OR: Joy DeGruy Publications; 2005 [cited 2020 Jul 26].

52. Rollnick S, Miller WR, Butler CC. Motivational interviewing in health care. New York: The Guilford Press; 2008.

53. Lundahl B, Moleni T, Burke BL, et al. Motivational interviewing in medical care settings: a systematic review and meta-analysis of randomized controlled trials. Patient Education Couns 2013;93(2):157–68.

54. Chair SY, Chan SWC, Thompson DR, et al. Long-term effect of motivational interviewing on clinical and psychological outcomes and health-related quality of life in cardiac rehabilitation patients with poor motivation in Hong Kong: a randomized controlled trial. Clin Rehabil 2013;27:1107–17.

55. Kabat-Zinn J, Massion AO, Kristeller J, et al. Effectiveness of a meditation-based stress reduction program in the treatment of anxiety disorders. Am J Psychiatry 1992;149:936–43.

56. Hofmann SG, Sawyer AT, Witt AA, et al. The effect of mindfulness-based therapy on anxiety and depression: a meta-analytic review. J Consult Clin Psychol 2010; 78(2):169–83.

57. Lau MA, Bishop SR, Segal ZV, et al. The Toronto Mindfulness Scale: development and validation. J Clin Psychol 2006;62(12):1445–67.

58. Shapiro SL, Brown KW, Thoresen C, et al. The moderation of Mindfulness-based stress reduction effects by trait mindfulness: results from a randomized controlled trial. J Clin Psychol 2011;67(3):267–77.

59. Shapiro S, Rechtschaffen D, de Sousa S. Mindfulness training for teachers. In: Schonert-Reichl K, Roeser R, editors. Handbook of mindfulness in education: mindfulness in behavioral health. New York: Spring; 2016. p. 83–97.

60. Association of Social Work Boards. About licensing and regulation. 2020. Available at: https://www.aswb.org/licensees/about-licensing-and-regulation/. Accessed July 12, 2020.

61. Association of state and Provincial psychology Boards. Licensure requirements. 2020. Available at: https://www.asppb.net/page/psybook. Accessed July 12, 2020.

62. Williams DR. Miles to go before we sleep: racial inequities in health. In: Valdez Z, editor. Beyond black and white: a reader on contemporary race relations. Los Angeles: Sage; 2017. p. 326–38.
63. Interprofessional Education Collaborative. Core competencies for interprofessional collaborative practice. 2011. Available at: https://www.ipecollaborative. org/resources.html. Accessed July 12, 2020.
64. Interprofessional Education Collaborative. Core competencies for interprofessional collaborative practice: 2016 update. 2016. Available at: https://www. ipecollaborative.org/resources.html. Accessed July 12, 2020.
65. McDaniel SH, Grus CL, Cubic BA, et al. Competencies for psychology practice in primary care. Am Psychol 2014;69(4):409–29.
66. Mauer BJ, Druss BG. Mind and body reunited: improving care at the behavioral and primary healthcare interface. J Behav Health Serv Res 2010;37(4): 529–42.
67. Davis TS, Guada J, Reno R, et al. Integrated and culturally relevant care: a model to prepare social workers for primary care behavioral health practice. Soc Work Health Care 2015;54:909–38.
68. Ashcroft R, McMillan C, Ambrose-Miller W, et al. The emerging role of social work in primary health care: a survey of social workers in Ontario family health teams. Health Soc Work 2018;43(2):109–17.
69. Fraher EP, Richman EL, de Saxe Zerden L, et al. Social work student and practitioner roles in integrated care settings. Am J Prev Med 2018;54(6):281–9.

Integrated Behavioral Health Role in Helping Pediatricians Find Long Term Mental Health Interventions with the Use of Assessments

Katie White, MA[a,*], Lydia Stetson, MA[a], Khadijah Hussain, BS[b]

KEYWORDS

- Integrated behavioral health • Assessment • Intervention • Mental health
- Pediatrics • Primary care

KEY POINTS

- Pediatricians are often the first to have contact with children and adolescents who may be impacted by developmental, behavioral, or mental health symptoms and can play a vital role in early intervention.
- Integrated behavioral health provides an important role in the primary care setting by assessing patients further and providing guidance for early intervention when concerns arise.
- Early intervention for any developmental, behavioral, or mental health condition can positively impact a person throughout their life.
- Using appropriate assessments is the cornerstone in identifying an accurate diagnosis, which can subsequently determine appropriate interventions.

INTRODUCTION

Pediatricians in the primary care setting are on the front lines in their contact and ability to recognize mental, developmental, and or behavioral health issues that are prevalent in pediatric patients; however, they often feel underequipped or unable to adequately diagnose, and subsequently treat, these problems owing to an insufficiency in training or a lack of time during appointments.[1–4] Because of this circumstance, mental health

[a] Division of Pediatric Psychology, Western Michigan University School of Medicine, 1000 Oakland Drive, Kalamazoo, MI 49008, USA; [b] MD Candidate Class of 2022, Western Michigan University Homer Stryker, MD School of Medicine, 1000 Oakland Drive, Kalamazoo, MI 49008, USA
* Corresponding author.
E-mail address: Kathryn.white@med.wmich.edu

Pediatr Clin N Am 68 (2021) 685–705
https://doi.org/10.1016/j.pcl.2021.02.006
0031-3955/21/© 2021 Elsevier Inc. All rights reserved.

pediatric.theclinics.com

concerns can be overlooked in the primary care setting, with earlier estimates indicating that nearly two-thirds of patients go undiagnosed, prompting a shift in awareness.[5,6] Studies have shown that early detection and treatment lead to better outcomes throughout a patient's life span and, if left untreated or inadequately treated, these symptoms can persist and lead to greater consequences over time.[4,7] For instance, research has suggested that if an adolescent's depression is not recognized and treated adequately, there are strong correlations with poor school performance, increases in substance abuse, and continual symptoms of depression into adulthood with suicide being one of the leading causes of death for this age group.[5] In 2004, the American Academy of Pediatrics developed a task force to determine ways pediatricians could heighten their understanding and ability to provide care for this population.[2] They estimated that mental health care would become a significant part of general pediatrics and their practice by 2020.[2] A result of the task force revealed a shortage of mental health clinicians in the primary care setting, which in turn led to the development of goals and guidelines for pediatricians to help bridge the gap between their ability to identify and manage mental health concerns, including ways to use assessments as way of detecting concerns.[6] Over the past decade, there has been a shift in the way primary care offices provide care, with a growing awareness of the benefits of having a multidisciplinary approach including working in conjunction with integrated behavioral health (IBH) clinicians.[3] A 2013 a study from Massachusetts determined that mild to moderate cases of common psychiatric disorders including anxiety, depression, and attention deficit hyperactivity disorder (ADHD) can be effectively managed in primary care offices; however, practitioners continue to feel inadequate in managing them.[4] IBH is highly valued by providers, and behavioral health integration programs can offer greater access to high-quality behavioral health services and resources by being implemented into pediatric primary care settings.[4] In many pediatric offices, IBH is implemented such that, when the clinician or screening tool identifies a behavioral health concern, an IBH clinician meets with the child and family to assess the patient further and figure out the next steps, including intervention or referral.[1]

CURRENT GUIDANCE FOR PRIMARY CARE PEDIATRICIANS

The early detection and treatment of behavioral health disorders have positive outcomes both with the patients and within the health care community, with accurate assessments being the cornerstone in identifying the disorder and subsequent delivery of appropriate interventions.[7,8] Developmental and behavioral disorders are considered to be 1 of the top 5 conditions causing impairment in functioning for children with behavioral and emotional problems identified as a leading cause of distress even if they do not meet the *Diagnostic and Statistical Manual of Mental Disorders*, 5th edition, criteria for a specific disorder.[9] Bright Futures and the American Academy of Pediatrics have developed guidance, recommendations, and policy statements on how, why, and when pediatricians can and should take steps in identifying and evaluating for developmental and behavioral health symptoms, including developmental screening, autism spectrum disorder screening, developmental surveillance, psychosocial and behavioral assessment, tobacco, alcohol and/or drug use assessment, and depression screening.[10–14] Table 1 offers a list of tools used in the pediatric primary setting to assess these various areas.[9,12,13,15,16] However, pediatricians continue to report barriers in their ability to provide screening and successful intervention with obstacles identified as often lacking the time needed to complete them, encountering long wait times and a lack of mental health providers for their patients to access

Table 1
Available assessments for use in pediatric primary care

Area	Tool	Details	Age	How to Obtain
Developmental Screener	Ages and Stages Questionnaire (ASQ-3)	Parent-completed questionnaire; series of 19–33 age-specific questionnaires screening communication, gross motor, fine motor, problem solving, and personal adaptive skills; results in pass/fail score for domains	4 mo–5 y	Paul H. Brookes Publishing Co: 800/638-3775; www.brookespublishing.com http://agesandstages.com/products-services/asqse-2
	Survey of Well-being of Young Children (SWYC)	Each form has sections on developmental milestones, behavioral/emotional development, and family risk factors. Autism-specific screening included at certain ages	1 mo–5 y	Free from website: https://www.floatinghospital.org/The-Survey-of-Wellbeing-of-Young-Children/Age-Specific-Forms
	Parents' Evaluation of Developmental Status (PEDS)	Single response form used for all ages, completed by parent (10 items); designed to screen for developmental and behavioral problems needing further evaluation; surveillance tool	0–8 y	Ellsworth & Vandermeer Press LLC: 888/729-1697; www.pedstest.com

(continued on next page)

Table 1
(continued)

Area	Tool	Details	Age	How to Obtain
Autism Spectrum Disorder Screening (autism spectrum disorder)	Modified Checklist for Autism in Toddlers (M-CHAT)	23-Item questionnaire completed by parent, designed to identify children at risk of autism	16–48 mo	Download: www.firstsigns.org/downloads/m-chat.pdf; Scoring: www.firstsigns.org/downloads/m-chatscoring.PDF
	Social Communication Questionnaire (SCQ)	40-Item questionnaire completed by parent, designed to identify children at risk of autism	≥4 y	Purchase: Western Psychological Services (www.wpspublish.com)
	Childhood Autism Spectrum Test (CAST)	Parent-completed questionnaire; 37 items; assess severity of autism spectrum disorder	4–11 y	https://www.autismresearchcentre.com/arc_tests https://psychology-tools.com/test/cast
	Pervasive Developmental Disorder Screening Test-II Primary Care Screener (PDDST-II PCS)	22-item questionnaire completed by parents to assess child's risk of autism	18–48 mo	Purchase: PsychCorp/Harcourt Assessment (www.harcourtassessment.com)

Psychosocial/ Behavioral Assessment	Vanderbilt ADHD Diagnostic Rating Scale	Completed by parent (55 items) or teacher (43 items). Elicits symptoms of inattention, disruptive behavior, anxiety, and depression; separate scale assesses functioning in school performance; includes a 26-item follow-up form	4–18 y	https://www.nichq.org/sites/default/files/resource-file/NICHQ_Vanderbilt_Assessment_Scales.pdf
	Pediatric Symptom Checklist (PSC-17)	Self-administered general psychosocial screening and functional assessment regarding attention, externalizing symptoms, and internalizing symptoms; 17 items completed by parent or youth >10 y	4–16 y	https://depts.washington.edu/hcats/FCAP/resources/PSC-17%20English.pdf
	Strength and Difficulties Questionnaire	Assesses 25 attributes divided into 5 scales. Completed by parent, teacher or youth 11–17 y; some versions include impact scale	3–17 y	https://www.sdqinfo.org/
	Adverse Childhood Experience Score	Measures childhood trauma using adverse childhood, community, and climate experiences; 10 items completed by parent; increasing scores associated with many adverse physical and mental health outcomes	Parent	http://acestoohigh.com/got-your-ace-score

(continued on next page)

Table 1
(continued)

Area	Tool	Details	Age	How to Obtain
Tobacco, Alcohol, or Drug Use Assessment	CRAFFT (Car, Relax, Alone, Forget, Friends, Trouble)	Youth interview or self-report; 3 screener questions followed by 6 items to assess for substance abuse	11–21 y	https://med.dartmouth-hitchcock.org/documents/CRAFFT-adolescent-substance-use-screen.pdf
	CAGE-AID	Youth self-report, 4 items used to screen for alcohol and drug abuse	Adolescent	https://www.hiv.uw.edu/page/substance-use/cage-aid http://www.agencymeddirectors.wa.gov/Files/cageform.pdf
Depression Screening	Patient Health Questionnaire Adolescent (PHQ-A)	PHQ-9 modified for teens; adolescent self-report designed to screen for depression	11–17 y	https://www.aacap.org/App_Themes/AACAP/docs/member_resources/toolbox_for_clinical_practice_and_outcomes/symptoms/GLAD-PC_PHQ-9.pdf
	Patient Health Questionnaire (PHQ-9)	Screens adults/adolescents for depression; 9 items; parent report	Parent/Adolescent	https://www.med.umich.edu/1info/FHP/practiceguides/depress/phq-9.pdf
	Kutcher Adolescent Depression Scale (KADS)	6, 11, or 16 items; self-report, designed to diagnose and assess the severity of depression	12–17 y	6-item: https://teenmentalhealth.org/wp-content/uploads/2014/09/6-KADS.pdf

Anxiety	Generalized Anxiety Disorder (GAD-7)	7 items plus impact scale (1 item) if positive responses; assesses for symptoms consistent with generalized anxiety disorder, or anxiety in patients with chronic disorders	11–17 y	https://www.mdcalc.com/gad-7-general-anxiety-disorder-7
	Screen for Child Anxiety Related Disorders (SCARED)	41 items, completed by parent or youth; assesses for anxiety but not obsessive-compulsive disorder or post-traumatic stress disorder	≥8 y	https://www.midss.org/content/screen-child-anxiety-related-disorders-scared
	Spence Children's Anxiety Scale (SCAS)	Parent or youth completed (35–45 items); assesses for anxiety including panic/agoraphobia, social anxiety, separation anxiety, generalized anxiety, obsessions/compulsions, and fear of physical injury	2–12 y	https://www.scaswebsite.com/1_1_.html

This table offers a list of tools, but is not meant to be an exhaustive list; rather, it is a representation of a range of the screenings that are available. Please refer to the Bright Futures Guidelines for Health Supervision of Infants, Children and Adolescents for more information on recommendations for health care professionals and for guidance on the use of these assessments.[10]

Abbreviation: PHQ, Patient Health Questionnaire 9.

support, concerns about liability, and seeing an increase in mandates for screening without extra time being allotted to do them while continuing to feel the pressure of being reimbursed.[9] As reported in **Table 1**, brief screener tools that take little time to implement and that do not require the expertise that other comprehensive instruments need, are available for pediatricians to use, although it is important to note that screening alone does not improve the outcomes for these patients.[7,8] Assessing children and adolescents can present with their own set of barriers in comparison to the adult population, which in turn makes it tricky to accurately identify a diagnosis.[8] To do this properly, a clinician must have the knowledge and training needed to complete a thorough assessment by gathering historical information regarding the youth's functioning in the various environments they inhabit.[8] They also require expertise and ability to dissect data from these assessment tools and integrate all of the information collected to render an accurate diagnosis.[8] An IBH clinician has the expertise and training needed to fulfill this requirement and is identified as a resource that can mitigate other barriers and concerns that pediatricians encounter when presented with a patient whom they are having a difficult time gauging.[4] Although there are a number of psychiatric, behavioral, mental health, and developmental disorders that a pediatric patient can be diagnosed with, for the purposes of this article, we focus on the IBH provider's role in further assessing identified concerns and their knowledge in providing appropriate interventions for ADHD, depression, developmental disorders, autism spectrum disorder, anxiety, and behavioral concerns.

THE ROLE OF INTEGRATED BEHAVIORAL HEALTH CLINICIANS IN ASSESSING BEHAVIORAL DISORDERS

Parents often discuss problems they encounter with their children and subsequently ask their child's pediatrician for suggestions on appropriate parenting techniques.[17] Between 37% and 39% of children will be diagnosed with a disorder, including a behavioral one, by the time they are 16.[17] An IBH clinician can help to triage the patient, assess the concerns presented, and in turn play a role in developing ways to target these behaviors.[17,18] Some of the most common behavioral complaints for children include symptoms of impulse control, disruptive behaviors, and oppositional and defiant behaviors.[9] Screening tools are available to assess for behavior symptoms in a primary care setting (see **Table 1**). However, a careful assessment for positive behavior symptoms is important. Assessors must consider the origin of the behavior and whether or not other issues are impacting its presence, including behavior and developmental disorders (ie, autism spectrum disorder), medical disorders (ie, somatic complaints), environmental factors (ie, victim of abuse or poor peer relationships), or caregiver factors (ie, inappropriate expectations or inadequate parenting techniques).[17] The IBH clinician can coordinate with pediatricians in delivering these tools and in providing further assessment when behaviors are identified. This practice can narrow down the symptoms to determine if the IBH professional can deliver brief interventions or whether a referral for longer term services or further psychological evaluation is needed. Various tools are listed in **Table 2**.

THE ROLE OF INTEGRATED BEHAVIORAL HEALTH CLINICIANS IN ASSESSING ATTENTION DEFICIT HYPERACTIVITY DISORDER

ADHD is the most common behavioral disorder reported in children and is described as a chronic condition that can affect academic performance, socialization, and overall health.[17] As reported in **Table 1**, physicians in a primary care setting can provide

Table 2
Additional tools available for IBH clinicians

Area	Tool	Details	Age Ranges	How to Obtain
Behavioral disorders	Behavior Assessment System for Children (BASC-3)	Assesses the behaviors and emotions of children (P and T)[a]	2–21:11 y	www.pearsonassessents.com
	Behavior Rating Inventory of Executive Function (BRIEF-2)	Screens for impairment in executive function (P, T, and S)[a]	5–18 y	www.parinc.com
	Beck Youth Inventories (BYI-2)	Self-report measure to assess for symptoms of depression, anxiety, anger, disruptive behavior and self-concept	7–18 y	www.pearsonassessents.com
ADHD	Brown Attention-Deficit Disorder Scales (Brown - ADD Scale)	Screen for and explore the executive and cognitive functioning associated with ADHD (P, T, and S)	3-adult	www.pearsonassessents.com
	Clinical Assessment of Attention Deficit (CAT-C)	Comprehensively assesses ADD/ADHD (P, T, and S)	8–79 y	www.parinc.com
	Conner's (Kiddie) Continuous Performance (K-CPT-2 and CPT-3)	Task-oriented computerized assessment of attention related problems	K-CPT-2 – 4–7 y CPT-3 - 8-adult	https://mhs.com
	Conners − 3	Tool used to measure ADHD associated with the *Diagnostic and Statistical Manual of Mental Disorders*, 5th edition, criteria (P, T, and S)	6–18 y	www.pearsonassessents.com
Depression	Children's Depression Inventory (CDI-2)	Self-report to assess cognitive, affective and behavioral signs of depression in children	7–17 y	www.pearsonassessents.com
	Reynolds Child Depression Scale (RCDS-2)	Self-report measures depressive symptoms in children	7–13 y	www.parinc.com
	Suicidal Ideation Questionnaire (SIQ and SIQ-Jr)	Self-report screener for suicidal ideation in adolescents	Grade 7–12	www.parinc.com

(continued on next page)

Table 2
(continued)

Area	Tool	Details	Age Ranges	How to Obtain
Anxiety	Multidimensional Anxiety Scale for Children (MASC-2)	Assesses the presence of symptoms related to anxiety disorders in youth	8–19 y	www.pearsonassessents.com
	Beck Anxiety Inventory (BAI)	Criteria referenced assessment for measuring anxiety severity level	17–80 y	www.pearsonassessents.com
	Revised Children's Manifest Anxiety Scale (RCMAS-2)	Measures the level and nature of anxiety as experienced by children	6–19 y	www.wpspublish.com
Developmental disorders/autism spectrum disorder	M-CHAT Follow up	A follow-up interview that is administered by a clinician when there is a positive M-CHAT screener	16–30 mo	https://m-chat.org
	Childhood Autism Rating Scale (CARS-2)	Uses direct observation to help distinguish between developmental delays in children who are not autistic with those that might be.	3–22 y	www.pearsonassessents.com
	Gilliam Autism Rating Scale (GARS-3)	Assessment of autism spectrum disorder and estimating severity level. (P and T)	3–22 y	www.pearsonassessents.com
	Adaptive Behavior Assessment System (ABAS-3)	Assesses adaptive skills and evaluates for concerns for developmental delays, autism spectrum disorder, intellectual disabilities, learning disabilities, neuropsychological disorders and sensory or physical impairments (P and T)	Birth – 89.11 y	www.pearsonassessents.com

This table offers a list of tools, but is not meant to be an exhaustive list; rather, it is a representation of a range of screenings available.
Abbreviation: ADD, attention deficit disorder.
[a] P, T, and S indicate that there are parent, teacher, and self-versions to assess the presence of symptoms across environments, respectively.

brief screeners when these concerns are presented; however, it is important for physicians to consider other factors that may account for the elevated symptoms, including an emotional or behavioral problem (ie, anxiety), developmental problem (ie, learning disorder), or a physical problem (ie, sleep disturbances).[17] IBH clinicians can help to facilitate further assessment to clarify the diagnosis by administering various assessments across caregivers in different environments (ie, home and school) or by administering a more in-depth, brief assessment in the office that can generate more specific data on ADHD symptoms. See **Table 2** for a list of additional tools. If ADHD is determined to be an appropriate diagnosis, the IBH professional can help physicians by describing the various treatments that are available along with their benefits and limitations (ie, medication and behavioral interventions) to the family.[17] If ADHD is not determined or is still questioned, the IBH professional can help to facilitate a referral to assess for a comorbid diagnosis or one that is better accounted for, as discussed elsewhere in this article.

THE ROLE OF INTEGRATED BEHAVIORAL HEALTH CLINICIANS IN ASSESSING DEPRESSION

Youth will likely experience depression at some point during adolescence, but it is often unidentified and untreated.[3] As stated elsewhere in this article and presented in **Table 1**, brief screeners are an efficient way to assess for symptoms.[8] However, they are not sufficient to substantiate a formal diagnosis and instead should prompt the use of a more comprehensive tool.[8] To render a diagnosis of depression, a thorough assessment needs to be completed and should include obtaining a family history of depression and a history of the patient's depression over time and across environments, completing assessments for comorbid disorders and assessing for suicidal ideation.[19] Although the completion of an in-depth evaluation may not be the role of an IBH clinician, they can help to gather some of these data in preparation to advocate for a more comprehensive psychological evaluation. They can also help to identify high-risk patients and provide information on an appropriate therapeutic intervention, in the interim of a full evaluation being completed.[20] **Table 2** lists some of the additional tools that IBH can use to help gather this information.

THE ROLE OF INTEGRATED BEHAVIORAL HEALTH CLINICIANS IN ASSESSING ANXIETY

Anxiety is one of the earliest symptoms to emerge in young children, affects 25% to 30% of children and adolescents, and is the most underidentified and undertreated of all disorders in this population.[9,21] Early detection is critical in preventing long-lasting poor outcomes into adulthood and in decreasing the risk of the emergence of depression, suicidality, substance abuse, medical problems, and disruptions to social and educational functioning.[21] **Table 1** provides some tools that can be used in the pediatric setting to assess for anxiety. Common anxiety disorders that frequently co-occur in this population are referred to as the "pediatric anxiety disorder triad," which includes generalized anxiety disorder, social anxiety disorder, and separation anxiety disorder.[22] Similar to depression, the role of the IBH clinician may not be to complete a full psychological evaluation, but they can help to gather further information for the child and family and provide more in-depth assessments to understand how anxiety is affecting the patient. This process can help to provide direction as to which therapeutic approach would be most beneficial. **Table 2** lists additional tools that IBH can complete.

THE ROLE OF INTEGRATED BEHAVIORAL HEALTH CLINICIANS IN ASSESSING DEVELOPMENTAL DISORDERS AND AUTISM SPECTRUM DISORDER

The earlier a developmental disorder, including autism spectrum disorder, is identified in a child, the better the prognosis over time.[12,13] Delays in obtaining a diagnosis can increase the risk for behavioral disorders or other developmental disorders.[12] **Table 1** lists some of the early screening tools used by pediatricians to assess for these symptoms. These disorders are often associated with a complicated criteria of symptoms that need to be met to qualify for a diagnosis. For example, the presentation of autism spectrum disorder symptoms and their severity can vary significantly across the spectrum, making it difficult to diagnosis the disorder accurately without a thorough evaluation.[13] Screeners such as the M-CHAT have been identified as the most widely used tools in primary care for screening for autism spectrum disorder and can help to discover potential symptoms.[23] However, it is also a tool that can have a high false-positive rate.[24] To detect these false positives, the M-CHAT follow-up interview plays a vital role.[24] However, there have been barriers identified in completing this portion of the assessment in the office, including difficulty reaching families for the follow-up interview and limitations in resources (ie, time and staffing) in a primary care setting.[24] These obstacles, along with the importance of completing the follow-up interview, suggests that it may be beneficial to conduct the interview immediately in the office when a positive screen is found.[24] Using an IBH clinician to facilitate this process is a useful way to capitalize on their expertise. As mentioned with other diagnoses, to officially qualify for an autism spectrum disorder diagnosis, a comprehensive assessment conducted by an interdisciplinary team with clinicians who have expertise in evaluating the symptoms of autism spectrum disorder (ie, child psychologists) is needed.[23] The IBH clinician can help to clarify a patient as an appropriate referral with by administering the additional assessments to help discern any false positives. It may be determined through these additional screeners that a more appropriate referral to specialists is required (ie, speech and language therapy, early on academic services). **Table 2** discusses other assessments that IBH can complete in the early detection of other developmental disorders.

CONCLUSION TO THE ROLE OF INTEGRATED BEHAVIORAL HEALTH CLINICIANS IN ASSESSMENT

Presenting concerns and all diagnosed disorders should be monitored over a child's lifespan to determine the effectiveness of and adherence to the treatment being provided (ie, therapeutic and/or medicinal).[17] The IBH practitioner can assist pediatricians in tracking this process by completing screeners at follow-up appointments, developing charts during the brief intervention appointments, and by asking parents and children how the presented symptoms have improved or worsened since interventions were introduced.[17] This practice can help pediatricians to adjust the level or the form of care being provided.

Beyond a primary care setting, the IBH clinician is a valuable and vital part of providing an optimal standard of care for patients in pediatric subspecialties and those with chronic medical conditions.[18,25] Suicide is the second leading cause of death in youth, with the risk being twice as high in those with chronic medical conditions.[25] Further, many other medical disorders incur an increased risk of depression, or other comorbid psychological, intellectual, adaptive, or behavioral conditions.[26,27] It is important to screen youth and adolescents for depression and other psychiatric and behavioral health disorders, because they can lead to a decreased health-related quality of life if left untreated.[26] The implementation of IBH as a part of an interdisciplinary team can improve a patient's overall quality of life and emotional functioning.[18]

THE USE OF ASSESSMENTS TO INFORM INTERVENTIONS

Mental health treatments, and subsequently IBH services, do not fit successfully into a one-size-fits-all model. Psychometric assessments are used to clarify presenting concerns as well as assist in determining the most appropriate course of action to follow. Because assessments can provide insight into the type of concern as well as the severity of the concern, assessments may then provide a guide to determining what type of intervention would be beneficial, what intensity of intervention is required, and how much time may be needed for the intervention to be efficacious. IBH is a method in which patients and families are provided mental health services quickly when concerns are identified by the primary care provider and that is cost effective.[28–30] Proximity to or the presence of mental health services within the primary care setting alone is insufficient to promote actual health care.[29] Thus, it is essential for IBH providers to not only be available, but also to have and be able to use tools to assist in the development of effective treatment plans and interventions. Integrated mental health clinicians, such as IBH providers, can provide a rapid assessment of mental health concerns and provide guidance or direct care services to the client or patient.[31] We will explore what interventions have been used within the IBH model and how these methods were chosen, in which cases referral to longer term treatment may be indicated, and potential methods for the use of psychometric assessments to determine the appropriate method, duration, and location of intervention for the presenting concern.

An important consideration with mental health interventions is whether the concerns are appropriate for brief, focused treatment, which may be offered by IBH services, or if longer term or more intensive treatment is required.[28] Bridges and colleagues[28] examined whether IBH providers chose interventions that were empirically based, appropriate to the patients' concerns, and whether the chosen interventions effectively predicted the rate of change for patients' concerns. Within IBH services in 2 primary care clinics, the most common diagnoses given to patients receiving IBH services included depression, anxiety, adjustment disorder, and childhood externalizing concerns, such as ADHD, oppositional defiance concerns, or conduct concerns.[28] Other participants in this study did not receive any specific mental health diagnosis, but rather were seen for life stressors or physical health concerns.[28] This study examined the evidence- based treatments that were provided and how the interventions aligned with the mental health diagnosis of the patient. The study found that, for patients with depressive concerns, the common interventions completed with IBH included behavioral activation and psychoeducation.[28] Patients with anxiety-related concerns received exposure therapy and relaxation training. Patients with adjustment disorder concerns were focused on behavioral activation and relaxation training.[28] Finally, patients with externalizing childhood concerns were commonly provided parent management training (PMT) or referral to an outside or non-IBH provider.[28] **Table 3** provides an overview of what evidenced-based interventions are commonly used for mental health concerns often seen in integrated health care settings.

THE USE OF BEHAVIORAL ACTIVATION IN INTEGRATED BEHAVIORAL HEALTH

Patients are most commonly referred to IBH services for concerns regarding depressive symptoms. Some research examines how evidence based treatment for depression or depressive symptoms may be adapted successfully for use in an IBH setting.[28,32] As typical IBH interventions are delivered in four to six 30-minute sessions, some adaptation of even brief focused therapies for depression are required

Table 3
Overview of interventions that may be used in IBH

Intervention	Presenting Concern	Details	Target Recipient
Acceptance and Commitment Therapy (ACT)	Workplace stress, test anxiety, social anxiety disorder, depression, obsessive-compulsive disorder, psychosis	Uses acceptance and mindfulness plus commitment and behavior change strategies to increase psychological flexibility (ie, being fully present in the moment, and either change or persist in behavior based on what the situation affords)	Individual experiencing stressors or condition
Behavioral Activation	Depression	Identification of specific goals that take the form of pleasurable activities that are consistent with the life one wants to live, and actively working toward those goals; designed to increase contact with positively rewarding activities; highly customizable and personalized	Individual with depression
Cognitive Behavioral Therapy (CBT)	Depression, anxiety, post-traumatic stress disorder, eating disorder, phobias	Make one aware of inaccurate or negative distortions in thought processes so that they can be countered and learn better ways of coping with problems; help view challenging situations more clearly and react to them in an effective manner	Patient with mental health disorder
Parent Management Training (PMT)	Parents of children with behavioral problems (such as ADHD or ODD) and are having trouble supporting or parenting them	Help to manage child's behavior and discipline child more effectively; learn strategies to correct negative, defiant behaviors	Parent/caregiver of younger children with ADHD or behavioral issues

| Relaxation *Training* | Anxiety; headache/chronic pain from chronic stressors | Bring about immediate stress relief and increased relaxation in therapy with training such as progressive muscle relaxation, breathing training, creative visualization, and mindfulness practice; can be used in conjunction with other cognitive behavioral techniques to aid stress relief; changes physiologic components of anxiety | Individual suffering from anxiety or other stressors |

This table offers a list of interventions, but is not meant to be an exhaustive list; rather, it is a representation of a range of interventions available.
Abbreviation: ODD, oppositional defiant disorder.

because these interventions are often composed of at least 14 sessions.[33] To modify behavioral activation to fit within a typical IBH timeframe, in this case 4 sessions plus a 12-week follow-up visit, the study described a sequence of intervention including first providing psychoeducation about the concern and setting an S.M.A.R.T. goal. The authors then described subsequent sessions as including review of any symptoms experienced and activities completed since the previous session; reviewing and adjusting goals or setting new goals as indicated by readiness for change; problem solving; and finally reviewing progress, problem solving, and making any necessary referrals to additional services.[32] The study found that the modified behavioral activation intervention was effective in decreasing depressive symptoms as measured by scores on the Patient Health Questionnaire 9 at baseline and at the 12-week follow-up.[32]

THE USE OF ACCEPTANCE AND COMMITMENT THERAPY IN INTEGRATED BEHAVIORAL HEALTH

Like behavioral activation, acceptance and commitment therapy (ACT) is an evidence-based treatment commonly used in the treatment of mental health concerns.[31] A retrospective study by O'Dell and colleagues[31] considered the use of modified ACT with adolescents in an integrated behavior health setting. The study found that the participants primarily had diagnoses, including ADHD, depression, adjustment disorder, conduct disorder, anxiety with adjustment disorders, depression, and anxiety being the most common. To examine symptoms and change in symptoms the participants were administered the Revised Children's Anxiety and Depression Scale.[31] After an average of 5.6 modified ACT sessions in an IBH setting, participants' scores on the Revised Children's Anxiety and Depression Scale showed significant improvement in symptoms of depression in particular.[31]

THE USE OF PARENT MANAGEMENT TRAINING IN INTEGRATED BEHAVIORAL HEALTH

Another concern often seen in IBH settings are childhood externalizing concerns such as ADHD, oppositional defiant disorder, and conduct disorder.[34,35] For such concerns, an intervention may include PMT, which is a broad term to describe interventions in which parents are taught skills that they can use to manage their child's behaviors.[34,35] As with other mental health treatment interventions, PMT is often administered over a period of time that is longer than the typical length or number of IBH sessions.[34] Gomez and colleagues[34] explored the question, "What actually happens when the BHC [behavioral health consultant] walks into a room with the patient and the patient's family?" The study described a procedure including triaging the patient and patient's family to determine if the patient and family were appropriate for IBH-based PMT or if referral to other providers was indicated.[34] The study reported that distress was measured using A Collaborative Outcomes Resource Network, which was given to parents as well as to the children as appropriate at the first and each subsequent behavioral health session.[34] The study found that the PMT modified for use in IBH was feasible and showed a significant change in distress level as measured by A Collaborative Outcomes Resource Network.[34]

THE ROLE OF INTEGRATED BEHAVIORAL HEALTH CLINICIANS IN INTERVENTIONS FOR AUTISM SPECTRUM DISORDER AND INTELLECTUAL OR DEVELOPMENTAL DISABILITY

Caregivers or parents of children with an autism spectrum disorder or intellectual or developmental disability may experience increased levels of caregiver stress, which can impact outcomes for not only the caregivers, but for the child as well.[36–38] One type of intervention that may be used to manage caregiver stress is mindfulness based interventions such as mindfulness-based stress reduction or ACT.[38,39] Although research suggests that using mindfulness-based interventions with the parents or caregivers of children with autism spectrum disorder and intellectual or developmental disability, there is limited research showing the effects of adapting mindfulness-based interventions for use in IBH.[38–40] Nonetheless, an IBH clinician may provide assessments for autism spectrum disorder and intellectual or developmental disability as well as screen for parental or caregiver stress and provide referrals as needed.

More intensive services for children with autism spectrum disorder often include early intensive behavioral intervention.[35,41] Early intensive behavioral interventions often require more time and greater use than would be feasible in IBH.[42,43] Therefore, the role of the IBH practitioner may be limited to assistance in the assessment of autism spectrum disorder before referring out to more intensive services. The IBH clinician may be able to assist, however, in providing supplemental problem-focused interventions on specific concerns, such as toileting concerns or specific problem behaviors.[41]

DETERMINING WHEN IT IS NECESSARY TO REFER BEYOND INTEGRATED BEHAVIORAL HEALTH SERVICES

It is important for providers to recognize that brief interventions provided by IBH providers may provide some relief of symptoms, but should not be viewed as a replacement for more intensive evidence-based treatment for mental health concerns requiring longer term treatment.[28,29] Bridges and colleagues[28] described in their study that patients requiring more than 6 sessions were coded as needing a referral to an outside provider rather than IBH services based on the provider's estimation of the severity of the presenting concerns. Referral for more intensive or outside providers would be appropriate for PMT when the concerns stemmed from parent or child psychopathology rather than concerns in parent and child interactions.[28] IBH services can be helpful because initiating treatment includes the primary care provider, who has likely already developed a rapport with the patient and their family and can thus provide a "warm handoff" from primary care to IBH services.[34] As seen in PMT, this warm handoff may occur and then the IBH provider may determine the appropriateness and type of services. Additionally, an IBH clinician may help patients to navigate the complexity of the health care system as patients move from childhood to adolescence to ultimately young adulthood.[44] Although the IBH clinician may not always provide the entirety of treatment, it is a beneficial step that may increase the accessibility of services and provide a service to patients that may not have otherwise been sought out.[30]

An IBH clinician can be advantageous in helping to determine what interventions may be effective and in providing these interventions as appropriate per the needs of the individual. The question at present asks how IBH services and primary care providers can most effectively and appropriately provide the necessary services as well as know when longer term services are required. As discussed elsewhere in this article, there has been research conducted on adapting traditional, evidence-based mental health interventions for use in IBH.[28,31,32,34] Additionally, as discussed elsewhere in this article, the IBH clinician can be used to assess for mental health concerns often seen in the primary care setting. Drawing from studies indicating the use of assessment by IBH, a sequence of services may include a triage or diagnostic interview, baseline assessment of presenting concerns by the parent or guardian as well as the child, determination of the method of intervention, and implementation of the intervention.[28] Additionally, assessments by IBH professionals may be used to track progress at specified points throughout the intervention, and IBH clinicians may conduct a follow-up assessment after the conclusion of the intervention. If the IBH provider determines that the scope of the presenting concerns is beyond what can appropriately be managed through IBH services, then they may refer to outside sources or specialty mental health care for more appropriate treatment. **Fig. 1** represents this proposed process.

CONCLUSION TO INFORMING INTERVENTION AND REFERRAL USING AN INTEGRATED BEHAVIORAL HEALTH ASSESSMENT

IBH providers may use assessments to determine when and if presenting concerns require more intensive services or referral to specialty mental health care services. The assessments completed by an IBH clinician may not only determine the type of intervention that constitutes the best practice for the presenting concern, but may also aid in determining when the severity of concerns falls beyond the scope of IBH services. Mental health concerns are dynamic and may change focus and grow or lessen in severity over time. Therefore, it is essential for IBH providers to be able to adapt to these changes. IBH professionals may thus use psychometric assessments to monitor for changes in the focus or severity of the presenting concerns to adapt to these changes and continue to provide effective services.

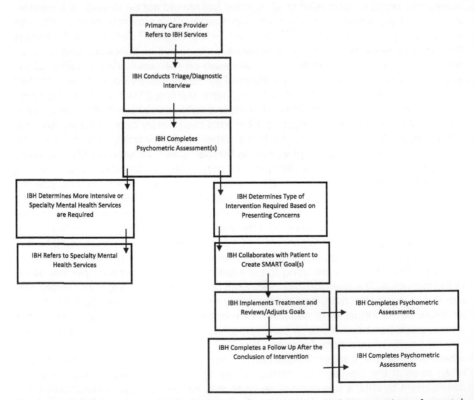

Fig. 1. Proposed sequence of IBH services in the assessment and intervention of mental health concerns presenting in primary.

CLINICS CARE POINTS

- Because primary care providers are usually first in line to identify concerns with developmental, behavioral, and/or mental health symptoms with their patient and are likely to have a long-standing rapport built with the families, there is a secure environment for a warm handoff to an IBH provider to address, support, and provide interventions.

- Two-thirds of patients in primary care settings have an undiagnosed disorder that likely impacts their functioning; providers often have insufficient training to identify them and lack time during appointments, which also impacts the primary care provider's ability to deliver suitable interventions.

- Studies have determined that mental health care is an important part of a general pediatric practice, which in turn supports the need for a multidisciplinary approach in providing the best system of care for their patients and families.

DISCLOSURE

There are no conflict of interests to disclose.

REFERENCES

1. Heinly MD, FAAP A, Bogus LCSW E, et al. Pediatric Primary Care and Integrated Behavioral Health. R Med J 2018;101(10):32–4. Available at: https://search.proquest.com/docview/2151200109?accountid=136549.
2. Foy JM. Pediatrics: introduction. Pediatrics 2010;125(SUPPL. 3):S69–74.
3. Cheung AH, Zuckerbrot RA, Jensen PS, et al. Guidelines for adolescent depression in primary care (GLAD-PC): II. Treatment and ongoing management. Pediatrics 2007;120(5):e1313–26.
4. Walter HJ, Vernacchio L, Trudell EK, et al. Five-year outcomes of behavioral health integration in pediatric primary care. Pediatrics 2019;144(1). https://doi.org/10.1542/peds.2018-3243.
5. Rinke ML, German M, Azera B, et al. Effect of mental health screening and integrated mental health on adolescent depression–coded visits. Clin Pediatr (Phila) 2019;58(4):437–45.
6. Zuckerbrot RA, Cheung A, Jensen PS, et al. Guidelines for adolescent depression in primary care (GLAD-PC): part I. Practice preparation, identification, assessment, and initial management. Pediatrics 2018;141(3). https://doi.org/10.1542/peds.2017-4081.
7. Mulvaney-Day N, Marshall T, Downey Piscopo K, et al. Screening for behavioral health conditions in primary care settings: a systematic review of the literature. J Gen Intern Med 2018;33(3):335–46.
8. Sattler AF, Leffler JM, Harrison NL, et al. The quality of assessments for childhood psychopathology within a regional medical center. Psychol Serv 2019;16(4):596–604.
9. Weitzman C, Wegner L, Blum NJ, et al. Promoting optimal development: screening for behavioral and emotional problems. Pediatrics 2015;135(2):384–95.
10. Hagan JF, Shaw JS, Duncan PME. Bright futures: guidelines for health supervision of Infants, children, and adolescents [pocket guide]. 4th edition. Elk Grove Village, IL: American Academy of Pediatrics; 2017.

11. Coleman WL, Dobbins MI, Garner AS, et al. Policy statement - The future of pediatrics: mental health competencies for pediatric primary care. Pediatrics 2009; 124(1):410–21.

12. Duby JC, Lipkin PH, Macias MM, et al. Identifying infants and young children with developmental disorders in the medical home: an algorithm for developmental surveillance and screening. Pediatrics 2006;118(1):405–20.

13. Johnson CP, Myers SM, Lipkin PH, et al. Identification and evaluation of children with autism spectrum disorders. Pediatrics 2007;120(5):1183–215.

14. Council on Community Pediatrics. Poverty and Child Health in the United States. Pediatrics 2016;137(4):e20160339.

15. Pediatrics AA of. Mental Health Tools for Pediatrics. Available at: https://downloads.aap.org/AAP/PDF/Mental_Health_Tools_for_Pediatrics.pdf#:~:text. The following table is a snapshot of a content can be integrated into pediatric primary care.

16. Sheldrick RC, Marakovitz S, Garfinkel D, et al. Comparative Accuracy of Developmental Screening Questionnaires. JAMA Pediatr 2020;174(4):366–74.

17. Hunter C, Goodie J, Oordt M, et al. Integrated behavioral health in primary care: step-by-step guidance for assessment and intervention. 2nd ed. American Psychological Association; 2017. https://doi.org/10.1037/0000017-000.

18. Rodríguez EM, Gulbas LE, George-Jones J, et al. Interdisciplinary perspectives on an integrated behavioral health model of psychiatry in pediatric primary care: a community-based participatory research study. Community Ment Health J 2019;55(4):569–77.

19. Hamrin V, Magorno M. Assessment of adolescents for depression in the pediatric primary care setting. Pediatr Nurs 2010;36(2):103–11. Available at: https://www.researchgate.net/publication/44605643. Accessed July 10, 2020.

20. Apple, RW; Patel, K; Smith, Z; White, K. The Role of Integrated Behavioral Health (IBH) in Suicide Prevention: Suicide and suicide prevention: A public health perspective Eds: Hatim Omar and Said Shahtahmasebi. Cambridge Scholar Publishing, Cambridge, United Kingdom (2019).

21. Rozenman M, Patarino KM. Pediatric anxiety in practice: a knowledge and needs. Assess Pediatr Nurses 2020;00(00):1–7.

22. Wehry AM, Beesdo-Baum K, Hennelly MM, et al. Assessment and treatment of anxiety disorders in children and adolescents. Curr Psychiatry Rep 2015;17(7). https://doi.org/10.1007/s11920-015-0591-z.

23. Kilmer M. Primary care of children with autism spectrum disorder. Nurse Pract 2020;45(6):33–41.

24. Khowaja MK, Hazzard AP, Robins DL. Sociodemographic barriers to early detection of autism: screening and evaluation using the M-CHAT, M-CHAT-R, and Follow-Up. J Autism Dev Disord 2015;45(6):1797–808.

25. Lois BH, Urban TH, Wong C, et al. Integrating suicide risk screening into pediatric ambulatory subspecialty care. Pediatr Qual Saf 2020;5(3):e310.

26. Guilfoyle SM, Monahan S, Wesolowski C, et al. Depression screening in pediatric epilepsy: evidence for the benefit of a behavioral medicine service in early detection. Epilepsy Behav 2015;44:5–10.

27. Soares N, Apple RW, Kanungo S. The role of integrated behavioral health in caring for patients with metabolic disorders. Ann Transl Med 2018;6(24):478.

28. Bridges AJ, Gregus SJ, Rodriguez JH, et al. Diagnoses, intervention strategies, and rates of functional improvement in integrated behavioral health care patients. J Consult Clin Psychol 2015;83(3):590–601.

29. Pomerantz AS, Kearney LK, Wray LO, et al. Mental health services in the medical home in the Department of Veterans Affairs: factors for successful integration. Psychol Serv 2014;11(3):243–53.
30. Hodgkinson S, Godoy L, Beers LS, et al. Improving mental health access for low-income children and families in the primary care setting. Pediatrics 2017;139(1). https://doi.org/10.1542/peds.2015-1175.
31. O'Dell SM, Hosterman SJ, Hostutler CA, et al. Retrospective cohort study of a novel acceptance and commitment therapy group intervention for adolescents implemented in integrated primary care. J Context Behav Sci 2020;16:109–18.
32. Funderburk JS, Pigeon WR, Shepardson RL, et al. Brief behavioral activation intervention for depressive symptoms: patient satisfaction, acceptability, engagement, and treatment response. Psychol Serv 2019. https://doi.org/10.1037/ser0000328.
33. Brief Behavioral Activation Intervention for Depressive Symptoms.pdf. BEHAVIOR MODIFICATION, Vol. 25 No. 2, April 2001 255-286 © 2001 Sage Publications, Inc.
34. Gomez D, Bridges AJ, Andrews AR, et al. Delivering parent management training in an integrated primary care setting: description and preliminary outcome data. Cogn Behav Pract 2014;21(3):296–309.
35. Ingersoll B, Straiton D, Caquais NRI. Role of Professional training experiences and manualized programs in ABA providers use of parent training with children with autism. Behav Ther 2020;51(4):588–600.
36. Neece CL, Green SA, Baker BL. Parenting stress and child behavior problems: a transactional relationship across time. Am J Intellect Dev Disabil 2012;117(1): 48–66.
37. Woodman AC, Mawdsley HP, Hauser-Cram P. Parenting stress and child behavior problems within families of children with developmental disabilities: transactional relations across 15 years. Res Dev Disabil 2015;36:264–76.
38. Dykens EM, Fisher MH, Taylor JL, et al. Reducing distress in mothers of children with autism and other disabilities: a randomized trial. Pediatrics 2014;134(2). https://doi.org/10.1542/peds.2013-3164.
39. Osborn R, Dorstyn D, Roberts L, et al. Mindfulness therapies for improving mental health in parents of children with a developmental disability: a systematic review. J Dev Phys Disabil 2020. https://doi.org/10.1007/s10882-020-09753-x.
40. Kanzler KE, Robinson PJ, McGeary DD, et al. Rationale and design of a pilot study examining Acceptance and Commitment Therapy for persistent pain in an integrated primary care clinic. Contemp Clin Trials 2018;66:28–35.
41. LeBlanc LA, Gillis JM. Behavioral Interventions for Children with Autism Spectrum Disorders. Pediatr Clin North Am 2012;59(1):147–64.
42. Yingling ME, Bell BA, Hock RM. Treatment utilization trajectories among children with autism spectrum disorder: differences by race-ethnicity and neighborhood. J Autism Dev Disord 2019;49(5):2173–83.
43. Vause T, Jaksic H, Neil N, et al. Functional behavior-based cognitive-behavioral therapy for obsessive compulsive behaviors in children with ASD: a randomized controlled trial.pdf. J Autism Dev Disord 2018;50:2375–88.
44. Babajide A, Ortin A, Wei C, et al. Transition cliffs for young adults with anxiety and depression: is integrated mental health care a solution? J Behav Heal Serv Res 2020;47(2):275–92.

Moving?

Make sure your subscription moves with you!

To notify us of your new address, find your **Clinics Account Number** (located on your mailing label above your name), and contact customer service at:

Email: journalscustomerservice-usa@elsevier.com

800-654-2452 (subscribers in the U.S. & Canada)
314-447-8871 (subscribers outside of the U.S. & Canada)

Fax number: 314-447-8029

Elsevier Health Sciences Division
Subscription Customer Service
3251 Riverport Lane
Maryland Heights, MO 63043

Printed and bound by CPI Group (UK) Ltd, Croydon, CR0 4YY

03/10/2024

01040401-0001